Machine Learning in Healthcare

Machine Learning in Healthcare

Fundamentals and Recent Applications

Bikesh Kumar Singh
G.R. Sinha

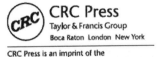

CRC Press
Taylor & Francis Group
Boca Raton London New York

CRC Press is an imprint of the
Taylor & Francis Group, an informa business

First edition published 2022
by CRC Press
6000 Broken Sound Parkway NW, Suite 300, Boca Raton, FL 33487-2742

and by CRC Press
2 Park Square, Milton Park, Abingdon, Oxon, OX14 4RN

CRC Press is an imprint of Taylor & Francis Group, LLC

Library of Congress Cataloging-in-Publication Data
Names: Singh, Bikesh Kumar, author. | Sinha, G. R., 1975– author.
Title: Machine learning in healthcare : fundamentals and recent applications /
Bikesh Kumar Singh, G.R. Sinha.
Description: First edition. | Boca Raton : CRC Press, 2022. |
Includes bibliographical references and index.
Identifiers: LCCN 2021042203 (print) | LCCN 2021042204 (ebook) |
ISBN 9780367564421 (hardback) | ISBN 9780367564438 (paperback) |
ISBN 9781003097808 (ebook)
Subjects: MESH: Machine Learning | Delivery of Health Care
Classification: LCC R855.3 (print) | LCC R855.3 (ebook) |
NLM W 26.55.A7 | DDC 610.285–dc23
LC record available at https://lccn.loc.gov/2021042203
LC ebook record available at https://lccn.loc.gov/2021042204

ISBN: 978-0-367-56442-1 (hbk)
ISBN: 978-0-367-56443-8 (pbk)
ISBN: 978-1-003-09780-8 (ebk)

DOI: 10.1201/9781003097808

Typeset in Times
by Newgen Publishing UK

Dedicated to my late father, Shri R. S. Singh Ji, and my PhD
joint supervisor, the late Dr. Kesari Verma
Bikesh Kumar Singh

Dedicated to my late grandparents, my teachers and Revered
Swami Vivekananda
G. R. Sinha

Contents

List of Figures...xiii
List of Tables..xvii
Preface..xix
Acknowledgments...xxiii
Author Bio xxv

Chapter 1   Biostatistics 1

    1.1   Data and Variables...1
    1.2   Types of Research Studies 2
    1.3   Sources of Medical Data..2
    1.4   Measures of Central Tendency.............................3
    1.5   Data Sampling and Its Types 5
        1.5.1   Probability Sampling Methods.................5
        1.5.2   Non-probability Sampling Methods..........6
    1.6   Statistical Significance Analysis 6
    1.7   Skewness...10
    1.8   Kurtosis 11
        1.8.1   Mesokurtic...13
        1.8.2   Leptokurtic 13
        1.8.3   Platykurtic 14
    1.9   Curve Fitting 14
        1.9.1   Linear and Non-linear Relationship 14
        1.9.2   Use of Curve-Fitting Method 14
    1.10   Correlation 14
        1.10.1   Pearson Correlation (PC)........................15
        1.10.2   Spearman Rank Correlation (SRC)..........16
    1.11   Regression...18
        1.11.1   Linear Regression....................................18
        1.11.2   Estimation of Regression Coefficients 19

Chapter 2   Probability Theory..23

    2.1   Basic Concept of Probability 23
    2.2   Random Experiment 24
    2.3   Conditional Probability..24
        2.3.1   Types of Events 25
    2.4   Bayes Theorem 26
    2.5   Random Variable..28
    2.6   Distribution Functions...28
        2.6.1   Binomial Distribution..............................29
        2.6.2   Poisson Distribution 30

	2.6.3	Normal Distribution 30
2.7	Estimation 31
2.8	Standard Error 32
2.9	Probability of Error 32

Chapter 3   Medical Data Acquisition and Pre-processing 35

3.1   Medical Data Formats...35
      3.1.1   Data Formats for Medical Images 35
            3.1.1.1   DICOM (Digital Imaging and
                      Communications in Medicine)...................36
            3.1.1.2   Analyse..36
            3.1.1.3   NIfTI (Neuroimaging Informatics
                      Technology Initiative) 36
            3.1.1.4   MINC (Medical Imaging NetCDF)............36
      3.1.2   Medical Data Formats for Signals.............................37
            3.1.2.1   EDF (European Data Format) 37
            3.1.2.2   BDF (BioSemi Data Format) 37
            3.1.2.3   GDF (General Data Format) 38
3.2   Data Augmentation and Generation...38
3.3   Data Labelling...38
3.4   Data Cleaning..39
      3.4.1   Statistical Approach..40
            3.4.1.1   Listwise Deletion 40
            3.4.1.2   Pairwise Deletion 40
            3.4.1.3   Multiple Imputation 40
            3.4.1.4   Maximum Likelihood Imputation.............41
      3.4.2   Machine Learning for Data Imputation......................41
            3.4.2.1   K-Nearest Neighbour (KNN).....................41
            3.4.2.2   Bayesian Network (BN).............................41
3.5   Data Normalization...42

Chapter 4   Medical Image Processing..45

4.1   Medical Image Modalities, Their Applications,
     Advantages and Limitations...45
      4.1.1   Radiography 46
      4.1.2   Nuclear Medicine 46
            4.1.2.1   Positron Emission Tomography (PET).......46
      4.1.3   Elastography...46
      4.1.4   Photoacoustic Imaging 47
      4.1.5   Tomography...47
      4.1.6   Magnetic Resonance Imaging (MRI)..........................47
      4.1.7   Ultrasound Imaging Techniques.................................48
4.2   Medical Image Enhancement...49
4.3   Basics of Histogram..51

4.4	Medical Image De-noising	56
	4.4.1	Spatial Filtering	56
		4.4.1.1 Linear Filters	56
		4.4.1.2 Non-linear Filters	58
	4.4.2	Transform Domain Filtering	58
		4.4.2.1 Non-data Adaptive Transform	58
		4.4.2.2 Data-Adaptive Transforms	59
4.5	Segmentation	59
4.6	Region-Based Methods	59
	4.6.1	Region-Growing Segmentation	61

Chapter 5 Bio-signals 65

5.1	Origin of Bio-signals	65
5.2	Different Types of Bio-signals	65
	5.2.1	Electrocardiogram	65
	5.2.2	Electroencephalogram (EEG)	68
	5.2.3	Electroocculogram (EOG)	69
	5.2.4	Electromyogram (EMG)	69
5.3	Noise and Artefacts	72
5.4	Filtering of Bio-signals	73
5.5	Applications of Bio-signals	74

Chapter 6 Feature Extraction 77

6.1	Feature Extraction	77
6.2	Echographic Characteristics of Breast Tumours in Ultrasound Imaging	78
6.3	Texture Feature Extraction	78
	6.3.1	First-Order Statistical Features	78
	6.3.2	Grey-Level Co-occurrence Matrices	82
	6.3.3	Grey-Level Difference Statistics	87
	6.3.4	Neighbourhood Grey-Tone Difference Matrix	88
	6.3.5	Statistical Feature Matrix	91
	6.3.6	Texture Energy Measures	92
	6.3.7	Fractal Dimension Texture Analysis	93
	6.3.8	Spectral Measures of Texture	95
	6.3.9	Run-Length Texture Features	96
6.4	Shape Feature Extraction	100
	6.4.1	Region Properties	100
	6.4.2	Moment Invariants	100
6.5	Feature Normalization	102
	6.5.1	Brief Overview of Feature Normalization Techniques	102

Chapter 7 Introduction to Machine Learning 107
    7.1 Introduction: What Is Machine Learning? 107
    7.2 Classification of Machine Learning (ML) Methods 108
    7.3 Steps in Implementation of Machine Learning 109
    7.4 Training, Testing and Validation 113
    7.5 Machine Learning Methods 114
        7.5.1 Supervised Learning 114
        7.5.2 Unsupervised Learning 125
    7.6 Performance Evaluation of Machine Learning Model 130

Chapter 8 Cancer Detection: Breast Cancer Detection Using
Mammography, Ultrasound and Magnetic Resonance
Imaging (MRI) 135
    8.1 Introduction 135
    8.2 Different Imaging Modalities 136
        8.2.1 Mammography (MG) 136
        8.2.2 Ultrasound (US) 137
        8.2.3 Magnetic Resonance Imaging (MRI) 140
    8.3 Breast Imaging Reporting and Data System
(BI-RADS) 141
    8.4 Usefulness of Machine Learning (ML) 141
        8.4.1 Image Pre-processing 142
        8.4.2 Image Segmentation 143
        8.4.3 Feature Extraction 143
        8.4.4 Feature Selection 145
        8.4.5 Classification 146
        8.4.6 Performance Evaluation 147
    8.5 Issues and Challenges 147
    8.6 Conclusion 149

Chapter 9 Sickle Cell Disease Management: A Machine Learning
Approach 153
    9.1 Introduction 153
    9.2 Severity Detection of Sickle Cell Disease 155
        9.2.1 Analysis of Clinical Complications 156
        9.2.2 Analysis of Clinical Attributes 156
        9.2.3 Analysis of Microscopic Images of RBC 158
    9.3 Hydroxyurea Dosage Prediction for SCD Patients 159
    9.4 Patient Response to Medications through
Hydroxyurea (HU) 165
    9.5 SCD Management Proposed Model 168
    9.6 Conclusions 168

Chapter 10   Detection of Pulmonary Disease 171

    10.1   Introduction to Pulmonary Disorders...................................... 171
    10.2   Restrictive and Obstructive Lung Diseases............................ 172
          10.2.1   Obstructive Lung Disease............................... 172
          10.2.2   Restrictive Lung Disease 173
    10.3   Diagnosis of Disease and Disorder 174
    10.4   Chest X-ray.. 175
    10.5   CT Scan 176
    10.6 S_pO_2 Level.. 179
    10.7   Arterial Blood Gas Analysis 180
    10.8   Laboratory Tests 180
    10.9   Bronchoscopy 181
    10.10 Sputum Test 182
    10.11 Pulmonary Function Test.. 183
    10.12 Challenges and Issues.. 185
    10.13 Application of Machine Learning in Diagnosis of
          Pulmonary Disorder.. 186
    10.14 Conclusion.. 188

Chapter 11   Mental Illness and Neurodevelopmental Disorders 191

    11.1   Neurodevelopmental Disorders... 191
    11.2   Developmental Dyslexia 191
          11.2.1   Diagnostic Methods.. 192
          11.2.2   Behavioural Method 192
          11.2.3   Brain Imaging Modalities............................... 193
          11.2.4   Recent Advancement in Diagnostic
                  Techniques 193
    11.3   Attention-Deficit/Hyperactivity Disorder (ADHD)............... 195
          11.3.1   Types 195
          11.3.2   Symptoms.. 195
          11.3.3   ADHD Screening 196
          11.3.4   Diagnosis Based on Brain Imaging and
                  Machine Learning Methods............................. 196
          11.3.5   Treatment for ADHD....................................... 197
    11.4   Parkinson's Disease 198
          11.4.1   Parkinson's Disease Prognosis and Measurement
                  Rating Scales 199
                11.4.1.1   HY Scale 199
                11.4.1.2   UPDRS Scale................................ 199
          11.4.2   Involvement of Digital Technologies for
                  Detection and Monitoring of PD 200
    11.5   Epilepsy.. 203
          11.5.1   Recent Literatures on Epilepsy Detection 203
          11.5.2   Generalized Machine Learning Model for
                  Epilepsy Detection System.................................... 204

11.6   Schizophrenia..205
       11.6.1   Recent Research..206
       11.6.2   A Machine Learning Model for Schizophrenia
                Detection 206

Chapter 12 Applications and Challenges..213

12.1   Role of Machine Learning in Healthcare Research..............213
12.2   Efficient Diagnosis of Diabetes...214
12.3   Neuropathy..215
12.4   Drug Monitoring 216
12.5   Bioinformatics..217
12.6   DNA Analysis 219
12.7   Digital Health Records...220
12.8   Future Research Challenges...221

Index..225

Figures

1.1   Steps involved in statistical analysis of data 7
1.2   Illustration of skewness 11
1.3   Illustration of skewness. (a) Negative skewed, (b) Normal (symmetric) and (c) Positive skewed 12
1.4   Illustration of kurtosis 13
1.5   An example of curve fitting 15
1.6   Scatter plots between variables "A" and "B" 16
1.7   Regression plot for variables x (independent) and y (dependent) 20
1.8   Severity of cancer patients' disease 20
2.1   Venn diagram representation of various types of events 26
2.2   Bayes theorem 27
2.3   Normal distribution bell curve 31
3.1   File formats for medical imaging 36
3.2   File formats for medical signals 37
3.3   Labelling process for supervised learning model 39
4.1   A typical block diagram of an ultrasound imaging system 48
4.2   Classification of image enhancement methods 49
4.3   Point processing of image enhancement 50
4.4   Masking operation 50
4.5   Image complement of a mammogram 51
4.6   Logarithmic transformation 51
4.7   Contrast enhancement 52
4.8   A typical histogram and histograms of images having different values of contrast 52
4.9   Histogram of input image 53
4.10   Histogram of output image after histogram equalization 54
4.11   An example of histogram equalization 54
4.12   Frequency domain operations 55
4.13   Various de-noising techniques used in medical image processing 57
4.14   Different segmentation techniques used in Image processing 60
4.15   Region-growing segmentation 61
4.16   (a) Original ultrasound image of benign breast, (b) Result of segmentation using FCM 62
4.17   (a) Original ultrasound image of benign breast, (b) Result of segmentation using k-means 62
5.1   A typical ECG waveform 66
5.2   ECG leads and Einthoven triangle 67
5.3   EEG 10–20 electrode placement 68
5.4   EEG bands 70
5.5   EOG signal [9] 71
5.6   EMG signal 72

6.1   Breast ultrasound image containing (a) malignant tumour and
       (b) benign tumour 79
6.2   Illustration of skewness. (a) Negative skewed, (b) Normal
       (symmetric) and (c) Positive skewed 81
6.3   Illustration of kurtosis. (a) Leptokurtic and (b) Platykurtic 82
6.4   The four orientations used to construct co-occurrence matrices 83
7.1   Different steps of machine learning 110
7.2   Division of labelled dataset 113
7.3   A support vector machine classifier 115
7.4   Non-linear support vector machine 116
7.5   Schematic of K-NN classifier for K = 3 and K = 5 117
7.6   Decision tree classifier (a) for binary data and (b) for numeric data 119
7.7   A random forest classifier with bagging 122
7.8   An artificial neural network model 123
7.9   Node function of an artificial neural network 124
7.10   (a) Scatter plot of data. (b) Data clusters 126
7.11   Confusion matrix representation 131
7.12   Representation of ROC-AUC curve 132
8.1   Different views used in mammography [6, 7] 136
8.2   Breast ultrasound images showing (a) Benign tumour
       (b) Malignant tumour [17] 138
8.3   Typical block diagram highlighting steps for breast cancer
       detection 142
8.4   Different types of image segmentation techniques 144
8.5   Commonly extracted type of features 145
8.6   Types of feature selection techniques 145
8.7   Different types of classifiers used in machine learning 146
8.8   Block diagram of implementation of the machine learning
       approach 148
9.1   ROC curve for different methods 157
9.2   Microscopic image of red blood cell 158
9.3   Circle Hough Transform method based normal and abnormal
       cell counting 159
9.4   Essential steps for Watershed segmentation 160
9.5   Experimental setup for dosage prediction 162
9.6   Experimental set-up and result for LSTM model 164
9.7   Experimental set-up for prediction of response for HU therapy 167
9.8   Proposed experimental setup for SCD management using
       machine learning 169
10.1   Types of pulmonary diseases 173
10.2   X-ray machine 176
10.3   Computer tomography machine 178
10.4   Pulmonary function test 184
10.5   Machine learning and image processing for diagnosis result
       of disorder 186

10.6   Signal processing using machine learning 187
11.1   Procedure involved in diagnosis of dyslexia and ADHD 194
11.2   Generalized block diagram of CAD system 201
11.3   Machine learning model for epileptic seizure detection system 205
11.4   Machine learning model for schizophrenia detection system 207
12.1   Classification of diabetes and required tests 214
12.2   Biomarkers used in diagnosis of diabetes 215
12.3   Drug monitoring and analysis 216
12.4   Different domains of bioinformatics 217
12.5   Various issues in bioinformatics 218
12.6   Tools used in analysis process 218
12.7   DNA analysis using machine learning 219
12.8   Electronic health records 220

Tables

1.1 Values and Their Mean Deviation 4
1.2 Results of Ten Students of a Class in Five Subjects 7
1.3 Results of Test of Normality 8
1.4 Parametric and Non-Parametric Test Comparisons 9
1.5 Two Sample *t*-test (Parametric Test) Result 9
1.6 Normality Test for Sickle Cell Patient Data 10
1.7 Result of Mann–Whitney *U* test 10
1.8 Age and Height of Young Girls 17
3.1 Feature Vectors x and Labels 39
3.2 Normalization Techniques and Formulas 42
8.1 Assessment Categories of BI-RADS 141
9.1 Clinical Attributes as Input Features 162
9.2 LSTM and ELM Performance Comparison 163

Preface

Artificial intelligence (AI) and machine learning (ML) methods have an increasing impact in our daily lives by enhancing the prediction and decision-making for the public in various fields like financial services, real estate business, consumer goods, social media and so on. However, despite several studies that have proved the efficacy of AI/ML tools in providing improved healthcare solutions, it has not gained the trust of health care practitioners and medical scientists. The primary reasons for this may be poor reporting on AI- and ML-based technologies, variability in medical data, the small size of data sets used, and a lack of standard guidelines for application of AI and ML in different domains of health and so on. Thus, substantial research is currently being conducted to establish AI and ML technologies as suitable for improving the public health. The development of new AI and ML tools for various domains of medicine is still an active field of research. Scientists from different fields like biomedicine, biotechnology, computer science, bioelectronics, information technology, mechanics (biomechanics) and materials (biomaterials) and so on are working together on the development and validation of new AI and ML tools to improve human health.

This book highlights and discusses how we can easily build various ML algorithms and how this can be applied to improve the healthcare system. AI and ML have various healthcare applications including in medicine, such as in medical data analysis, early detection and diagnosis of diseases, in providing objective-based evidence to reduce human error, reducing inter- and intra-observer errors, in risk identification and interventions for management of human healthcare, real-time health monitoring, continuous health monitoring, in assisting clinicians and patients in selecting appropriate medications, identifying and evaluating drug response and so on.

WHAT THE BOOK DOES FOR THE READER

The present book offers an extensive demonstration and discussion on various principles of machine learning and its application in healthcare. An effort is made to first expose the readers to fundamental concepts, which include mathematical requisites and the traditional machine learning framework. Then, traditional and advanced machine learning methods and their applications in the broad medical field are presented. Solved examples are given to extend the understanding of the reader along with exercises.

WHO SHOULD READ THIS BOOK?

This book is for readers who are willing to understand machine learning without any background knowledge and are further looking to implement a healthcare system based on machine learning models. The readers of this book are expected to be students, faculty and scientists who are interested in learning about and applying machine learning tools to solve real-life problems. Though the book may be beneficial for students, faculty and scientists from all domains, we have especially focused on healthcare-related applications. In fact, the contents of the book are presented so that it can be suitable for both self-study and classroom teaching.

WHY WE WROTE THIS BOOK

There are many books on machine learning and AI. However, there are limited books which start from the basics of machine learning and cover its application to the healthcare system. This is in stark contrast to how machine learning is being used, as a commodity tool in research and healthcare applications. We hope this book will help people who want to apply machine learning to the healthcare system.

A brief summary of all the chapters of the book is as follows. The contents of this book are divided into three parts. The first part provides necessary background for unfamiliar readers. For readers, who are naive, necessary mathematical prerequisites and background concepts are provided in Chapters 1–3. The role of statistical methods and probability is important in solving real-time problems, Chapters 1 and 2 are included to provide fundamentals of these topics. Chapter 3 introduces data recording and data pre-processing principles. Since medical images and bio-signals play a crucial role in health analytics, a brief overview of the same is presented in Chapters 4 and 5. These two chapters discuss medical imaging modalities and the basics of bio-signal origin, followed by their important characteristics and clinical significance. Algorithms to de-noise signals and images are then presented.

The second part of the book is dedicated to traditional machine learning techniques and their applications. This part is divided into two chapters (Chapters 6 and 7). Chapter 6 introduces some popular feature extraction techniques from medical images. Chapter 7 introduces machine learning architecture and explains basic terminologies useful for readers in understanding advanced-level chapters later in the book. Once medical data is recorded as images or signals, the next step is to represent data as appropriate quantitative variables/features. Chapter 7 also presents traditional machine learning techniques. Each algorithm is explained step by step and solved examples are provided to give confidence to the readers so that they may use them in solving their own research problems. Some computational simulations are also provided for immediate application and understanding. The advantages and limitations of different algorithms are also discussed, though traditional machine learning techniques have their own utility in solving research problems with limited data sets and computational resources.

After exposing the readers to fundamental and advanced-level concepts of machine learning, some popular applications of machine learning techniques are presented in part 3 of this book, which includes five chapters (Chapters 8–12). Applications investigated by the authors of this book and also those by other researchers are presented. Each chapter (Chapters 8–12) starts with emphasis on the importance of the issue followed by how machine learning tools were applied to address the issue. Applications like computerized diagnosis/management of cancer (Chapter 8), sickle cell disease (Chapter 9), pulmonary disorders (Chapter 10), diseases related to mental health (Chapter 11) and finally, some other important applications of machine learning in the management of diseases like diabetes, hypertension and drug monitoring and their challenges are also discussed (Chapter 12).

This book attempts to bring fundamental and advanced concepts of machine learning under one roof along with a comprehensive list of applications and case studies. The authors would be happy to receive comments that would be helpful in improving the contents of the book.

Acknowledgments

Dr. Bikesh K. Singh expresses his heartfelt thanks to mother, Shrimati Renu Devi, his wife, Pushpanjali Singh, and his two sons, Shourya and Reyansh, for their uncondi-tional and continuous support during the completion of this book, *Machine Learning in Healthcare: Fundamentals and Recent Applications*. Their wonderful support and encouragement throughout the completion of this important book have been a great strength. The blessings of his late father, Shri R. S. Singh Ji, have always been an inspiration for the book.

Dr. Bikesh is extremely thankful to his PhD scholars, Anurag Shrivastava, Divya Singh, Hardik Thakkar, Kushangi Atrey, N. P. Guhan Seshadri, Soumya Jain, Sunandan Mandal and Yogesh Sharma, for their help and support throughout the tenure of writing this book.

This book is the outcome of sincere efforts that could be given to the book only due to the great support of family members, and therefore Dr. Sinha expresses his gratitude and sincere thanks to his family members, his wife, Shubhra, his daughter, Samprati, and his parents and teachers.

Dr. Singh expresses his thanks to the director of his institute, NIT Raipur, and also extends his sincere thanks to the directors of MIIT Mandalay Myanmar and IIITB Bangalore for their encouragement and support.

We would like to thank all our friends, well-wishers and all those who keep us mo-tivated in doing more and more, better and better. We sincerely thank all contributors for writing relevant theoretical background and real-time applications of *Machine Learning in Healthcare*.

We express our humble thanks to Dr Gagandeep Singh, publisher (Engineering) and all editorial staff of CRC Press for their great support, necessary help, appreci-ation and quick responses. We also wish to thank CRC Press for giving us this oppor-tunity to contribute on a relevant topic with a reputed publisher. Finally, we want to thank everyone, in one way or another, who helped us in editing this book.

Last but not least, we would also like to thank God for showering us with his bless-ings and strength to do this type of novel and quality work.

Bikesh Kumar Singh
G. R. Sinha

Author Bio

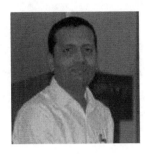

Dr Bikesh Kumar Singh is Assistant Professor in the Department of Biomedical Engineering at the National Institute of Technology Raipur, India, where he also earned his PhD in biomedical engineering. He has 21 years of teaching experience, and for five years he served as the head of the Department of Biomedical Engineering. He has published more than 70 research papers in various international journals and conferences. He is the recipient of the Chhattisgarh Young Scientist Award, the IETE Gowri Memorial Award and the IEI Young Engineer Award.

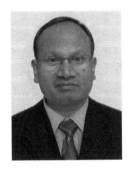

Dr G. R. Sinha is Adjunct Professor at the International Institute of Information Technology Bangalore (IIITB) and deputed as Professor at Myanmar Institute of Information Technology (MIIT) Mandalay Myanmar. He was a visiting professor (Honorary) in Sri Lanka Technological Campus Colombo during 2019–2020. He was a visiting professor for teaching a short graduate course on cognitive science and brain computing research at the University of Sannio, Italy, during September 2020–March 2021.

He has published 280 research papers, book chapters and books at the international level that include *Biometrics* (Wiley India); *Medical Image Processing* (Prentice-Hall of India); and 13 edited books. He is associate editor of five SCI/Scopus-indexed journals. He has 23 years of teaching and research experience. He has been dean of faculty and executive council member of Chhattisgrah Swami Vivekak and Technical University and is currently a member of the Senate of MIIT. Dr Sinha has been delivering Association of Computing Machinery (ACM) lectures as ACM Distinguished Speaker in the field of Digital Signal Processing since 2017 across the world. A few of his more important assignments include expert member for the Vocational Training Program by Tata Institute of Social Sciences (TISS) for Two Years (2017–2019); Chhattisgarh Representative of Institute of Electrical and Electronics Engineers MP Sub-Section Executive Council (2014–2017); distinguished speaker in the field of digital image processing by the Computer Society of India (2015). He served as distinguished IEEE lecturer in the IEEE India council for the Bombay section.

He is the recipient of more than 12 awards and recognitions at national and international levels. He has delivered more than 50 keynote/invited talks and chaired many technical sessions in international conferences across the world, such as Singapore,

Myanmar, Sri Lanka, Irvine (California), Italy and India. He is consultant for various skill development initiatives of National Skill Development Corporation, Government of India. He is a regular referee of project grants under the Department of Science and Technology-Extra Mural Research scheme and several other schemes of the government of India.

1 Biostatistics

LEARNING OBJECTIVES

This chapter aims to cover:

- Importance of biostatistics
- Description of the most important biostatistics used in analysis and classification of biomedical and medical applications
- The role of statistics in mathematical modelling

In the last decade, interest in mathematical modelling and analysis of underlying phenomena in the diverse field of biology have significantly grown. This includes the design of experiments and the formulation of the research hypothesis, sources of biological and medical data, data collection methods, analysis, and interpretation and evaluation procedures. The broad field which encompasses all these steps is termed biostatistics. Biostatistics deals with development of statistical techniques for analysing data associated to living organisms. The purpose of this chapter is to present an overview of fundamental concepts in biostatistics and its application in health research.

1.1 DATA AND VARIABLES

Data includes variables, observations or measurements obtained from elements of the population. "The population" means the group considered for study, for example, someone who wants to study possible risk factors that may lead to cancer in the future. In this situation, the study population will comprise cancer patients and the risk factors will be measurements recorded from these patients. Data or the collection of data is sometimes also referred to as a database. There are several ways of categorizing data, and the data can be qualitative or quantitative, discrete or continuous, nominal or ordinal and so on. Let's understand these concepts with some examples.

Consider the female breast cancer risk prediction problem using certain variables such as dietary habits (vegetarian/non-vegetarian), smoking habits (yes/no), waist size, hip size, waist-hip ratio (WHR), socio-economic status (low, middle, high), body mass index, number of children and number of abortions. Here, variables such

DOI: 10.1201/9781003097808-1

as dietary habits, smoking habits and socio-economic status are qualitative variables as these cannot be expressed as a number, while other variables, namely age, waist size, hip size, waist-hip ratio (WHR), body mass index and routine blood pathology measures are quantitative as these variables can be represented as numbers. Quantitative variables can be further classified into continuous or discrete, and continuous variables can take any numeric value, and discrete variables can take only a finite number of values. For example, waist size, hip size, waist-hip ratio (WHR) are continuous variables, while variables such as number of children and number of abortions are discrete. The third category, is the nominal or ordinal subcategory of qualitative variables. The variables dietary habits and smoking habits are nominal variables as these variables are not ordered. On the other hand, variables such as socio-economic status, which can be ordered in series or sequence, are called ordinal.

1.2   TYPES OF RESEARCH STUDIES

Data required in various research studies is sometimes available from past events (retrospective study) or the collection of the data is required from future events/patients (prospective study). The former is less time-consuming; however, it is subject to recall bias. Recall bias is an error caused due to difficulty in recalling past events or information, resulting in less accurate, less reliable and incomplete data. In a retrospective study, the participants can be interviewed about their past exposure/illness. Other examples include examining old medical records (medical images, biomedical signals, clinical opinions, pathology etc.), old research manuscripts or newspaper or magazine articles that have highlighted the variables needed. Examples of a prospective study include interviewing and physically examining the participants, analysing pathological tests, questionnaires and so on during subsequent follow-ups throughout the period of study.

1.3   SOURCES OF MEDICAL DATA

Once you formulate the research question to be answered, the next step is to figure out the types and sources of data needed to generate the score and hence answer your question. This section deals with various sources of health data. The data collected can be either primary or secondary depending upon whether it is collected directly from the subjects or the data used is collected by someone else respectively. Health data sources primarily include health surveys, administrative/claims data and medical records/electronic health records of subjects, surveillance, wearable devices, disease registries, vital records, open source, clinical trials and research articles.

- Health surveys from subjects are conducted generally through questionnaires and interviews through emails, telephonic conversations or in one-to-one meetings. Examples of surveys in health research include, the National Health Interview Survey, the National Immunization Survey, the National Centre for Health Statistics survey and so on.
- Administrative data is the data different government/public agencies or other organizations gather about their operations and services towards patient care.

It includes bills, insurance details, patients' registration/appointments, service delivery and so on.

- A medical record (or electronic health record) includes information about the medical history of the patient and care given. Information such as diagnosis, pathology reports, treatment procedures, medications recommended and so on can be extracted from the electronic health records of patients.
- Clinical trial data is initiated from voluntary participation in a diseased and healthy population study. Data collection takes place for the defined duration of study followed by its processing and analysis.
- Vital records include information such as births, details of birth, death and its cause, death-causing diseases and foetal mortality. In the United States, the National Vital Statistics System is one such example of how the vital data of their population is provided.
- In the last few years, research on the design of wearable devices like smart watches has gained significant attention. Such devices can be used for continuous analysis of human activity and human vital signs which can be helpful in remote monitoring of patients.
- Open-source repositories like the UCI Machine Learning Repository (https://archive.ics.uci.edu/ml/index.php), PhysioNet (https://physionet.org/), the Cancer Imaging Archive (https://www.cancerimagingarchive.net/) and so on are increasingly becoming popular as source of data for health and machine learning research.
- Currently, many peer-reviewed articles and their authors have studied the research data obtained through experimental study design, survey or various other study methodologies. There has been a substantial increase in research journals which publish research data – including its recording protocols, demographics of participants, and ground truth validations – which can be useful for other scientists to validate their own methodology and results.

1.4   MEASURES OF CENTRAL TENDENCY

In statistics, central tendency indicates the centre point or value at the central position of the whole dataset. This is usually the first step in statistical analysis and is useful in understanding the characteristics of overall data in a summarized way. The three main measures of central tendency are mean, median and mode.

Mean: Summation of the value of every observation in a dataset divided by the total number of observations is called arithmetic mean or arithmetic average. Mathematically, it is defined as:

$$\mu = \frac{\sum_{i-1}^{M} n_i}{M},$$

(1.1)

where μ is the mean, n_i represents the value of different observations, and N is the total number of observations.

TABLE 1.1
Values and Their Mean Deviation

Values	21	22	21	24	24	25	90	100
Deviation from mean	−19.875	−18.875	−19.875	−16.875	−16.875	−15.875	49.125	59.125

The mean indicates the most common observation, and the advantage of using the mean is that its calculation comprises all the observations in the dataset and that the sum of deviations from each value from the mean is always zero. Further, the mean can be used for both a continuous as well as a discrete-valued dataset. However, it is affected by values which are unusual or uncommon (also called outliers) in the dataset. Table 1.1 shows an example of some values and deviations from the mean values.

Solved Example 1.1: Calculate the mean of the following values: 21, 22, 21, 24, 24, 25, 90, 100. Prove that the sum of deviations from each value from the mean is always zero. Also comment on the effect of outliers.

$$\text{Solution : Mean} = \frac{21+22+21+24+24+25+90+100}{8} = 40.875$$

Now, let's calculate the deviation of different observations from the mean (*deviation = values-mean*):

$$\text{Sum of deviations} = -19.875 - 18.875 - 19.875 - 16.875$$
$$-16.875 - 15.875 + 49.125 + 59.125 = 0$$

It can also be observed that the mean (= 40.875) may not be the best representative of given data because most of the data given lies between 21 and 25 (90 and 100 being outliers). Thus, additional measures of the central tendency are required.

Median: The central point of the data arranged in ascending or descending order is called the median. The advantage of the median measure is that it is less influenced by outliers. The number of data points above and below the median is the same. It is calculated in the following way:

- In case the number of datapoints is odd, the median is the value at the exact centre of the data after arranging them in either ascending or descending order. For example, the median of {2, 1, 3} will be 2.
- In case the number of data points is even, the median is the average of the two middle numbers in the data after arranging them in either ascending or descending order. For example, the median of {2, 1, 4, 3} will be the average of 2 and 3, that is, 2.5.

Solved Example 1.2: Given the following numbers: 1, 8, 10, 2, 4, x, 7, 3, 9, if x is the median, find the possible value(s) of x.
Solution: Since x is the median value, that is, the central value, if the given numbers are arranged in ascending or descending order, it will exactly lie at the centre. Thus,

The ascending order of the given numbers: {1, 2, 3, 4, x, 7, 8, 9, 10}. Thus, the possible values of x can be 5 or 6.

Mode: The value or the number with the highest occurrence in the data is called its mode. For example, the mode of dataset {5, 3, 3, 7, 8} is 3 as 3 occurs twice, while the others occur only once.

Solved Example 1.3: Given the following numbers: {1, 2, 1, 3, 2, 3, 3, 2, 2, 5, 1, 6, 8, 3}, find its mode.
Solution: Since numbers 2 and 3 both appear four times, the mode is 3 and 4.

1.5 DATA SAMPLING AND ITS TYPES

When conducting research, the collection of data from the whole population being studied is impractical. However, it is possible to study the whole population by its subset and thus, sampling can be defined as the collection of a data/sample representing the larger population being studied. The sampled data must be representative of the population to confirm the generalization of research outcomes to the population in totality. Sampling methods are broadly classified as those based on probability and those without any probability. Let us learn about some popular sampling methods.

1.5.1 PROBABILITY SAMPLING METHODS

In probability sampling, there is equal probability to choose each sample in the population, and this is also called random sampling. Probability sampling results in a generalized result due to which it is regarded as the best method to study a representative subset; however, these are more time-consuming than non-probability sampling. Probability sampling can be conducted with and without replacement. In probability sampling with replacement, the sample, once considered, is returned to the population and the population size remains unchanged throughout the data collection. In contrast, in probability sampling without replacement, the sample, once selected, is not returned to the main population. Thus, the population size goes on reducing as the sampling continues. The other types of probability sampling methods are:

Systematic sampling – Samples are chosen at steady intervals after arranging all the samples in a specific order. The required sample size defines the interval. Assume that a systematic sampling of 100 lung cancer patients from such 1,000 admitted to hospital in a year is required to study their vital signs. Then, each patient can be numbered serially as 1, 2, ..., 1000, and every tenth (*Note that interval = 1000/ 100 = 10*) patient can be considered as a sample (10, 20, 30, 40......., 100, 110, 120, ..., 1000). If the starting point is different, that is, one can start with the second patient, the selected samples will be different (2, 12, 22, 32, 42, 52, ...1092).

- *Stratified sampling* – This sampling technique is used when the population being studied is heterogeneous. The whole population is split into different groups called *strata* based on some prior knowledge of sample characteristics. All the samples corresponding to particular *strata* share common characteristics. An equal number of samples are taken from each group to conduct the study. For instance, consider the previous example of sampling of 100 lung cancer patients out of 1,000. We may consider stratifying the population by cancer type or stage, and then an equal number of samples can be obtained from each group through random sampling.

1.5.2   NON-PROBABILITY SAMPLING METHODS

Non-probability is non-random sampling, wherein the study does not consider the whole sampling population, leaving some samples with no probability of being selected. The results of non-probability sampling usually cannot be generalized; however, this method is convenient and less time-consuming. One of the popular non-probability sampling methods is purposive sampling.

- *Purposive sampling* – Samples based on the researcher's judgement are selected without using any specific technique. This approach is less time-consuming and is convenient; however, it is subject to errors and bias due to the individual's judgement.

1.6   STATISTICAL SIGNIFICANCE ANALYSIS

Statistical analysis of data refers to the procedure of data interpretation, prediction of trends and the pattern from data using different statistical operations. There are different types of statistical analysis of data: descriptive analysis, inferential analysis, prescriptive analysis, predictive analysis and so on. The first two are the main types of statistical data analysis. The descriptive statistical analysis of data is based on simply analysing the central tendency and measure of spread in the data, whereas, in the case of inferential statistical data analysis, parameter estimation and a hypothesis test are used to generalize the data. For statistical analysis, Statistical Analysis System (SAS), R software, MedCalc software, MATLAB and Statistical Package for the Social Sciences (SPSS) are a few of the various statistical software packages available to perform statistical tests. The aim of this section is to explain the steps involved for inferential statistical analysis of data based on the data type. This section of the chapter also explains the method for identifying the distribution of the population using a normality test. Based on the distribution of the population, parametric or non-parametric tests are applied for statistical analysis. We try to explain the steps involved for deciding the type of data and selecting the best-fit test using examples. Many parametric and non-parametric tests are available based on the data type. However, this section covers *two sample t-test*s and *ANOVA* (analysis of variance) under the parametric test category and the *Mann–Whitney* U *test* under the non-parametric test category as these are the most commonly used. Figure 1.1 shows the steps to perform statistical analysis of data.

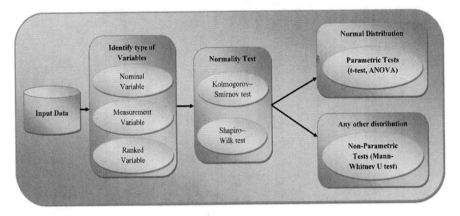

FIGURE 1.1   Steps involved in statistical analysis of data.

TABLE 1.2
Results of Ten Students of a Class in Five Subjects

Student Name	Result (Pass/Fail)	Position in Class	Marks				
			Subject 1	Subject 2	Subject 3	Subject 4	Subject 5
Student 1	Pass	1	94	92	86	90	83
Student 2	Pass	2	87	90	82	84	76
Student 3	Pass	3	80	76	82	77	81
Student 4	Pass	4	69	72	81	71	70
Student 5	Pass	5	69	65	64	63	71
Student 6	Pass	6	68	61	50	54	52
Student 7	Fail	7	30	40	41	45	46
Student 8	Fail	8	31	25	33	37	29
Student 9	Fail	9	25	30	15	25	40
Student 10	Fail	10	15	12	07	22	20

Variable Type: To decide the statistical test, the first step is to identify the variable type. Usually the variables are classified into three categories: nominal variable, measurement variable and ranked variable. To understand this, let us consider an example shown in Table 1.2. The table shows the results of ten students in a class. The second column of the table shows the overall results of the student whom I either pass or fail is actually the nominal variable because here the observations are classified into discretized categories, that is, pass or fail. The third column of the table is the position of the student in that class from one to ten. It is a ranked variable, also known as an ordinal variable. The variables from columns 4 to 8 consist of marks obtained by the students in different subjects, which is the measurement variable, also called the scaled variable.

Normality Test: The next step for statistical analysis is to test the normality of the data, and based on the normality test results, parametric or non-parametric tests are

TABLE 1.3
Results of Test of Normality

Subject	Result	Kolmogorov-Smirnov[a]			Shapiro-Wilk		
		Statistic	df	Sig.	Statistic	df	Sig.
Subject1	Fail	.242	4	.	.870	4	.299
	Pass	.289	6	.127	.858	6	.182
Subject 2	Fail	.190	4	.	.991	4	.962
	Pass	.197	6	.200*	.916	6	.476
Subject 3	Fail	.217	4	.	.939	4	.649
	Pass	.352	6	.019	.803	6	.062
Subject 4	Fail	.251	4	.	.925	4	.564
	Pass	.125	6	.200*	.982	6	.959
Subject 5	Fail	.206	4	.	.968	4	.831
	Pass	.256	6	.200*	.884	6	.287

applied. For the assessment of normality, there are two different ways: first by using the graphical method and second by assessing numerically. In the case of a lack of graphical judgement, it is better to rely on numerical assessment. Table 1.3 shows the results of a test of normality for the above example from the Shapiro-Wilk Test and the Kolmogorov-Smirnov Test. The Shapiro-Wilk Test works well with a small sample size, whereas the Kolmogorov-Smirnov Test performs well with a large sample size. The confidence interval considered is 95%. The significant value (p-value) in the Shapiro-Wilk test (in the last column) is more than 0.05, which confirms that the data is normally distributed and the parametric test should be used. If the p-value is less than 0.05, then it shows that the data is not normally distributed and non-parametric tests needs to be applied.

Parametric and Non-parametric Test: A parametric or non-parametric test is selected based on the distribution of population. Table 1.4 shows a brief comparison of parametric and non-parametric tests and some of the tests from each category.

Parametric Test: For data considered in Table 1.2, a parametric test is applied. For the nominal variable and the measurement variable, a two-sample t-test and ANOVA both can be applied. The student's t-test for the two samples is mathematically identical to a one-way ANOVA with two categories. Here, the data consist of two categories: pass or fail. So, the two-sample t-test is applied and the result is shown in Table 1.5. From the result, it is clear that the significant value (p-value) for both the categories of data is less than 0.05, which indicates that there is a significant difference in the means of the two categories, as also indicated in the table. Hence the measurement variables are statistically associated with the nominal variable for the two categories.

Non-parametric Test: To apply and understand the non-parametric test, a pathological dataset of a sickle cell patient is considered in this study. The data consists of

TABLE 1.4
Parametric and Non-Parametric Test Comparisons

Non-parametric Test	Parametric Test
Does not require data to follow normal distribution. **Distribution-free tests**	Requires data to follow normal distribution
Nonparametric analyses to assess group medians	Parametric analyses to assess group means
• 1-sample sign • Mann–Whitney test • Kruskal-Wallis	• 1-sample t-test • 2-sample t-test • One-way ANOVA

TABLE 1.5
Two Sample t-test (Parametric Test) Result

Subject	t	df	Sig. (2-tailed)	Mean Difference	Std. Error Difference
Subject 1	8.338	8	.000	52.58333	6.30634
	9.086	7.979	.000	52.58333	5.78708
Subject 2	6.177	8	.000	49.25000	7.97375
	6.304	7.025	.000	49.25000	7.81212
Subject 3	5.275	8	.001	50.16667	9.51105
	5.150	6.050	.002	50.16667	9.74138
Subject 4	5.105	8	.001	40.91667	8.01556
	5.361	7.571	.001	40.91667	7.63262
Subject 5	5.261	8	.001	38.41667	7.30148
	5.220	6.404	.002	38.41667	7.35914

827 samples with two types of variables. The first type of variable is the nominal variable. Here the data consists of four different complications in a patient: icterus, cyanosis, lymphadenopathy and haemolytic face. Each complication has two categories of value, yes: when a complication is present, and no when it is not present. The second type of variable is the measurement variable, which here is the percentage value of sickle haemoglobin (HbS). The normality test has been conducted in the data and it shows that the p-value is less than 0.05 for all the complications in both the categories, as shown in Table 1.6.

Hence the data is not normally distributed, so the Mann–Whitney U test is applied to the data, as shown in Table 1.7. The result shows that the p-value for icterus, lymphadenopathy and haemolytic face is less than 0.05 and for cyanosis it is more than 0.05. Hence, the conclusion can be drawn that the three complications: icterus, lymphadenopathy and haemolytic face, are statistically associated with HbS levels, whereas cyanosis is not statistically associated with HbS levels.

TABLE 1.6
Normality Test for Sickle Cell Patient Data

Haemoglobin variant		HbS	
Test		Kolmogorov-Smirnova	Shapiro-Wilk
Complications	Class	Sig.	Sig.
Icterus	0	.000	.000
	1	.000	.000
Cyanosis	0	.000	.000
	1	.000	.000
Lymphadenopathy	0	.000	.000
	1	.000	.000
Haemolytic face	0	.000	.000
	1	.000	.000

TABLE 1.7
Result of Mann–Whitney U test

Complications	p-value (Hbs)
Icterus	.000
Cyanosis	.286
Lymphadenopathy	.000
Haemolytic face	.000

1.7 SKEWNESS

Skewness is a statistical measure which is defined as the estimate of asymmetry present in the probability distribution of any random variable around its mean value. In other words, it tells us about the lack of symmetry in the distribution. It can take any value, that is, positive, negative, zero or infinite.

The Pearson formula to calculate skewness is given below:

$$Skewness = E[(X - \mu)^3]/\sigma^3, \tag{1.2}$$

where

μ : stands for mean,
σ : stands for standard deviation,
X : stands for random variable and
E is the statistical expectation.

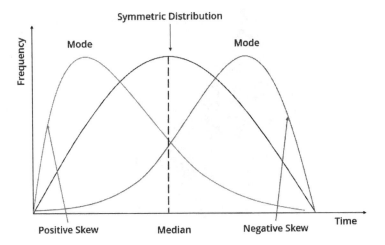

FIGURE 1.2 Illustration of skewness.

For a symmetric distribution like a Gaussian distribution which gives a bell-shaped curve, the measure of skewness is zero. In this case the tail of the curve on both sides of the central tendency measure is even, and so they balance each other giving a zero value of skewness. But in the case of asymmetrical distribution, the shape of the graph is inclined towards either the left or the right side where one side of the tail is long and thin and other side is short and fat. Thus, we can categorize the skewness in two types: *positive skewness* and *negative skewness*. Below, Figures 1.2 and 1.3 illustrate this clearly. For positively skewed data, the tail is shifted towards the right side, and for the negatively skewed data, the tail is shifted towards the left side of the median. To understand this more clearly, let us take an example. Consider a dataset of the marks scored by students on a test. Suppose the test was easy, so the marks scored by students range from 30 to 90 and most of the students scored above 65. In this case, the central tendency is 50, so the graph indicating the distribution of marks will be tilted towards the right and the tail is on left side because it is skewed towards the left side (negatively skewed) as the maximum of the scored marks of students higher than the central measure. Now suppose the test was conducted again and this time the test was very tough and the maximum students scored lower than 45. In this case, the graph will be tilted towards the left side and the tail is on the right side (positively skewed) as most of the students scored lower than the central measure (median).

1.8 KURTOSIS

The word "kurtosis" is derived from the Greek word *kyrtos* or *kurtos*, which means curved. Kurtosis is a statistical measure which tells us about the "tailedness" of a distribution. Sometimes it is misinterpreted as the "peakedness" of the distribution. Kurtosis describes the shape of the distribution curve's tail at its extreme values with respect to the median or central tendency measure. It is also called the Pearson fourth moment regarding its mean.

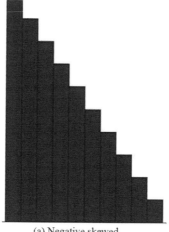

(a) Negative skewed

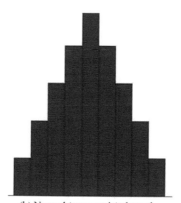

(b) Normal (symmetric) skewed

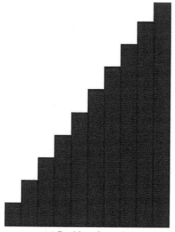

(c) Positive skewed

FIGURE 1.3   Illustration of skewness. (a) Negative skewed, (b) Normal (symmetric) and (c) Positive skewed.

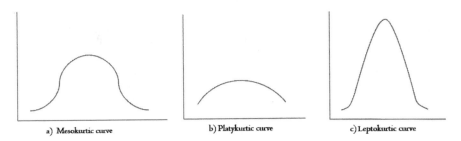

a) Mesokurtic curve
b) Platykurtic curve
c) Leptokurtic curve

FIGURE 1.4 Illustration of kurtosis.

The Pearson formula to calculate kurtosis is given below:

$$Kurtosis = E[(X - \mu)^4]/\sigma^4, \tag{1.3}$$

where

μ: stands for mean,
σ: stands for standard deviation,
X: stands for random variable and
E is the statistical expectation.

A bell-shaped curve depicting the normal distribution has a kurtosis value 3. Hence we can calculate the excess kurtosis value of a distribution with respect to the normal distribution by using the formula:

$$Excess\ kurtosis = Kurtosis - 3. \tag{1.4}$$

Excess kurtosis can take any value, be it be positive, negative or zero. Depending upon these values, kurtosis can be categorized into three types: *mesokurtic, leptokurtic*, and *platykurtic*. Below, Figure 1.4 shows the different curves of various distributions.

1.8.1 MESOKURTIC

The data distribution having an excess kurtosis value of zero or near zero is called mesokurtic distribution. Its curve shows a medium peak value, and the mesokurtic distribution follows the normal distribution; therefore, it is considered as the reference for other distribution.

1.8.2 LEPTOKURTIC

The data distribution having an excess kurtosis value as positive is called leptokurtic distribution. Its curve shows a sharp peak and heavy tails which are near to the median value. Extreme positive value indicates that maximum observations are located in the tails portion and not around the central tendency measure.

1.8.3 PLATYKURTIC

The data distribution having an excess kurtosis value as negative is called as platykurtic distribution. Its curve shows very dispersed flat peaks and light tails which are far from the median value. Extreme negative value indicates that fewer observations are located in the tails portion and maximum observations are located around the central tendency measure.

1.9 CURVE FITTING

The curve-fitting method is the process of finding a mathematical relation and modelling a curve that provides the best fit for the given data points, or in simple words, this method is used to find an appropriate curve that characterizes the most approximate plot close to the original series of data points. It involves interpolation, extrapolation and smoothing of the given data points to form the best-fit curve. These curves are used as very powerful tools to visualize the data and to predict the behaviour of a function where no data points are available.

In regression analysis the method of approximation of the given data to a relationship of certain parameters with the aid of mathematical expression and equation is called curve-fitting analysis. It can be also defined as the method of interpreting the curve with the given dataset on a curve that most suitably fits its shape and provides a best-fit curve for the analysis of the parameters. It also allows us to find the relationship between different parameters responsible for getting such a curve and their relationship with each other too. Below, Figure 1.5 shows an example of curve fitting and approximation.

1.9.1 LINEAR AND NON-LINEAR RELATIONSHIP

The curve the relationship between the independent variable and dependent variable is non-linear in nature, or it cannot be uniform throughout the domain. With a unit change in the independent variable, the change in the dependent variable is not constant throughout the entire domain; rather, it is region dependent.

1.9.2 USE OF CURVE-FITTING METHOD

It is sometimes very difficult to find the non-linear relationship with only graphical values and datasets, so to obtain such a relation the curve-fitting method is used, which gives us a best-fitted curve for a given set of data points because the dataset can be easily analysed and understood by visualizing it in the form of a graph.

1.10 CORRELATION

Correlation is a tool used to define "how strong is the degree of relationship" between two random variables. The relationship between the two variables "A" and "B" can be in two ways, namely, 1) with the incremental variable "A," the value of variable "B" also tends to increase (positive slope); 2) with the incremental variable "A," the

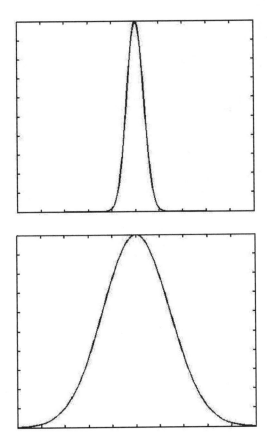

FIGURE 1.5   An example of curve fitting.

value of variable "B" also tends to decrease (negative slope). The former is known as positive correlation while latter is termed as negative correlation. Figure 1.6 displays these two kinds of relationships graphically. The strength of the correlation is defined by the correlation coefficient, generally represented by Greek letter ρ.

The two popular correlation schemes, namely, Pearson correlation and Spearman rank correlation are extensively used in data research methodologies for the optimization of parameters and the justification of results statistically. Brief descriptions of both schemes are given in the below subsections.

1.10.1   PEARSON CORRELATION (PC)

This is also known as the "Pearson product-moment correlation" between two random variables "A" and "B." Its value varies between −1 to +1. Mathematically, the Pearson correlation coefficient is defined as:

$$\rho_{A,B} = \frac{cov(A,B)}{\sigma_A \sigma_B},$$ (1.5)

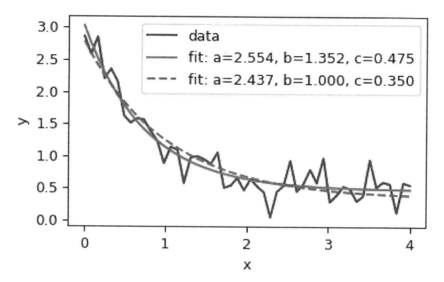

FIGURE 1.6   Scatter plots between variables "A" and "B" showing positive (left graph) and negative (right graph) correlation.

where $\mathrm{cov}(A, B)$ is the covariance between variables "A" and "B," and σ_A and σ_B are the standard deviation of variables "A" and "B" respectively.

If variables "A" and "B" belong to a sample consisting n values, then Equation (1.6) can be represented as:

$$\rho_{A,B} = \frac{\sum_{i=1}^{n}\left(A_i - \overline{A}\right)\left(B_i - \overline{B}\right)}{\sqrt{\sum_{i=1}^{n}\left(A_i - \overline{A}\right)^2}\sqrt{\sum_{i=1}^{n}\left(B_i - \overline{B}\right)^2}}, \qquad (1.6)$$

where A_i and B_i are i^{th} sample values, and $\overline{A}$ and $\overline{B}$ are sample means.

If $\rho_{A,B} = +1 \rightarrow$ strong positive correlation.
If $\rho_{A,B} = -1 \rightarrow$ strong negative correlation.
If $\rho_{A,B} = 0 \rightarrow$ no correlation between "A" and "B."

PC follows certain assumptions on the distribution of data. It assumes that both variables are drawn from a normal distribution with homogeneous variance. Therefore, it is also known as the Pearson parametric correlation test.

1.10.2   Spearman Rank Correlation (SRC)

Unlike the Pearson correlation, the Spearman correlation is a non-parametric test that does not make any assumptions about the data distribution. Here, the variables are

TABLE 1.8
Age and Height of Young Girls

Age (in yrs)	Height (in cm)
6	63
10	72
8	75
12	77
5	58

first aligned corresponding to their ranks in the distribution. In other words, SRC is nothing but the PC computed on the ranks of two non-parametric random variables. Mathematically, the SRC coefficient is defined as:

$$\text{Spearman } \rho_{rA,rB} = \frac{\text{cov}(rA, rB)}{\sigma_{rA}\sigma_{rB}}, \tag{1.7}$$

where rA and rB are the ranks of the two random variables "A" and "B."

If there are m different ranks belonging to two random variables then, the SRC coefficient can be represented according to the following simple formula:

$$\text{Spearman } \rho_{rA,rB} = 1 - \frac{6\sum d_r^2}{m(m^2 - 1)}, \tag{1.8}$$

where d_r is the difference between the ranks of two random variables for each observation.

Exercise 1: Let us assume that the age and height of five young girls are as shown in Table 1.8.

To check whether these two variables have any significant relationship, we compute Pearson and Spearman rank correlation coefficients.

1) Calculation of Pearson correlation coefficient

A	H	$(A - \bar{A})$	$(A - \bar{A})^2$	$(H - \bar{H})$	$(H - \bar{H})^2$	$(A - \bar{A})$ $(H - \bar{H})$
6	63	−2.2	4.84	−6	36	13.2
10	72	1.8	3.24	3	9	5.4
8	75	−0.2	0.04	6	36	−1.2
12	77	3.8	14.44	8	64	30.4
5	58	−3.2	10.24	−11	121	35.2
Mean $(\bar{A}) = 8.2$	Mean $(\bar{H}) = 69$		$\Sigma = 32.8$		$\Sigma = 266$	$\Sigma = 83$

From Equation (1.5),

$$\rho_{A,H} = \frac{83}{\sqrt{32.8} \times \sqrt{266}} = 0.88.$$

The coefficient value (positive and close to +1) indicates that there is a significant relation between the age and height of the young girls.

2) Calculation of Spearman rank correlation coefficient

Let us assume that the top rank is given to the highest value for both the variables.

A	H	Rank A	Rank H	d_r	$(d_r)^2$
6	63	4	4	0	0
10	72	2	3	−1	1
8	75	3	2	1	1
12	77	1	1	0	0
5	58	5	5	−0	0
Mean $(\overline{A}) = 8.2$	Mean $(\overline{H}.) = 69$				$\Sigma = 2$

From Equation (1.8),

$$Spearman\ \rho_{rA,rH} = 1 - \frac{6 \times 2}{5(5^2 - 1)} = 0.9.$$

Hence, the SRC also shows a strong positive relation between the two variables.

1.11 REGRESSION

Regression analysis is a process in which the value of the target variable is determined on the basis of prediction variables. The target variable is also known as the dependent variable, whereas the predictors are known as the independent variables. There are several types of regressions. In this chapter, we discuss briefly linear regression and its estimation.

1.11.1 LINEAR REGRESSION

This is the simplest form of regression analysis. The dependent variable is generally of a continuous nature, and there is a linear relationship between dependent and independent variables. If there is one target variable and only one predictor, then the regression is known as simple linear regression, whereas if there are more than one predicting variable, the regression is called multiple linear regression. The expression of linear regression with more than one predictor is represented as:

$$y = a_0 + a_1 x_1 + a_2 x_2 + a_3 x_3 + \dots\dots + a_n x_n, \tag{1.9}$$

where $a_0, a_1 \dots a_n$ are regression coefficients.

1.11.2 ESTIMATION OF REGRESSION COEFFICIENTS

Let us take a simple linear regression model equation, for example:

$$y = a_0 + a_1 x_1. \tag{1.10}$$

The primary task is to deduce the values of coefficients a_0 and a_1. According to the least-square model, the coefficients are determined by the following equations [2]:

$$a_1 = \frac{\sum_{i=1}^{n} \left(x_i - \bar{x}\right) \left(y_i - \bar{y}\right)}{\sum_{i=1}^{n} \left(x_i - \bar{x}\right)^2} \text{ and } \tag{1.11}$$

$$a_0 = \bar{y} - a_1 \bar{x}, \tag{1.12}$$

where $\bar{x}$ and $\bar{y}$ are the mean of variables x and y respectively.

Exercise 2: Let the columns of Table 1.8 be considered variables x and y, where x is the independent variable and y is the dependent variable.

x	Y	$(x - \bar{x})$	$(x - \bar{x})^2$	$(y - \bar{y})$	$(x - \bar{x})(y - \bar{y})$
6	63	−2.2	4.84	−6	13.2
10	72	1.8	3.24	3	5.4
8	75	−0.2	0.04	6	−1.2
12	77	3.8	14.44	8	30.4
5	58	−3.2	10.24	−11	35.2
Mean ($\bar{A}$) = 8.2	Mean ($\bar{H}$) = 69		Σ = 32.8		Σ = 83

Therefore, from Equations (1.11) and (1.12),

$$a_1 = \frac{83}{32.8} = 2.53 \text{ and } a_0 = 69 - \left(2.53 \times 8.2\right) = 48.25.$$

So, the required expression for a simple linear regression (from Equation (1.10)) will be:

$$y = 48.25 + 2.53x_1. \tag{1.13}$$

Figure 1.7 shows the scatter plot of variables x and y along with their regression line given by Equation (1.13). From Figure 1.8, it is evident that the regression line satisfactorily fits the variable events.

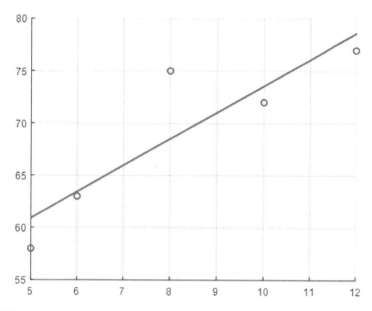

FIGURE 1.7   Regression plot for variables x (independent) and y (dependent).

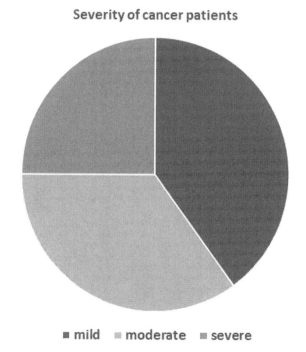

FIGURE 1.8   Severity of cancer patients' disease.

1.12 LEARNING OUTCOMES

After studying this chapter, students will be able

- to apply appropriate statistics in biomedical applications for the analysis and evaluation of results.

Let us further understand the concepts of the variables with the following two questions.

Question 1.1: Classify the following variables as: (a) quantitative or qualitative; (b) continuous or discrete; (c) nominal or ordinal:
Blood group, volume of tumour, ethnic origin, entropy of a matrix, electrocardiogram (ECG), QRS amplitude, power in EEG bands, intelligence quotient (IQ) score, blood pressure, body temperature, number of patients discharged in a week, haemoglobin.

Question 1.2: The pi-chart shown in Figure 1.8 illustrates the severity of cancer patients in admitted hospital "X" for a specific period of time. What type of data does it show?

2 Probability Theory

LEARNING OBJECTIVES

This chapter aims to cover:

- Basics of probability
- Types of probability functions

2.1 BASIC CONCEPT OF PROBABILITY

A probability denotes a number that further indicates the chance of occurrence of any particular event. Probability theory is a branch of mathematics which deals with the number of possibilities and likelihood of any event to occur. For any event, the value of probability lies between zero and one. Zero value of probability indicates that there is 0% chance of the event occurring and this event is called an impossible event. On the other hand, when the value of probability is one, it means there is 100% chance of an event occurring and this event is called a certain event. A probability of 0.50 means out of 100, there is a 50% chance of the event occurring. Let us take an example to understand this. Suppose a fair die is rolled. Then chance of getting a number greater than seven is 0%, whereas the chance of getting a natural number is 100% because any fair die will have only natural numbers between one and six. Now let us consider the classic example of tossing a coin where we will have only two possibilities, which are getting a head or a tail. Since both events are equally likely, the probability of getting a head on a single toss thus is 50%.

The probability can be mathematically expressed as the ratio of the possible outcomes of an event happening to the total number of outcomes that can happen in a random experiment.

$$\textit{Probability of an event} = \frac{\textit{number of ways an event can occure}}{\textit{total number of outcomes}} \quad \dots \quad (2.1)$$

DOI: 10.1201/9781003097808-2

2.2   RANDOM EXPERIMENT

A random experiment can be defined as an experiment whose outcomes cannot be predicted with certainty. An experiment is said to be deterministic if it has only one outcome, and is called random if it has more than one outcome. If an experiment has exactly two outcomes, then it is called a Bernoulli trial. If the outcomes cannot be determined before the experiment is performed, then it is said to be a random experiment.

As discussed above, random experiments have a number of possible outcomes that define the probability of a certain event to happen. Before proceeding further, let us discuss some definitions related to probability and random experiment.

Sample space: The set of all possible results of a random experiment.
Event: The set of event outcomes fulfilling certain conditions.
Favourable outcomes: The number of results that fulfil the necessary condition
    of a desired outcome of an event.
Trial: The number of times an event is performed.

Let us make all the above definitions with an example:

Solved Example 2.1: A fair coin is tossed three times. Determine the following

    i.   Sample space.
    ii.   Number of trials.
    iii. Probability of getting only one head.
    iv.   Probability of getting at most two tails.

$$\underline{\text{Solution}}\text{: Sample space(S)= }\{(HHH)(HHT)(HTH)(THH)(HTT)$$
$$(THT)(TTH)(TTT)\} \dots \qquad \text{(i)}$$

$$\text{Number of trials = number of time experiment is performed = 3} \dots \qquad \text{(ii)}$$

Probability of getting only one head = Event 1 =$\{(HTT)(THT)(TTH)\}$

Therefore, the number of favourable outcomes = 3

The probability of getting only one head = 3/8 ... $\qquad$ (iii)

Probability of getting at most two tails = Event 2 =$\{(HHH)(HHT)(HTH)(THH)$
$$(TTH)(THT)(HTT)\}$$

Therefore, the number of favourable outcomes = 7

The probability of getting at most two tails = 7/8 ... $\qquad$ (iv)

2.3   CONDITIONAL PROBABILITY

It is defined as the probability of occurrence of an event when one preceding event has already occurred. This type of probability involves the happening of two events one after the other. For understanding such complex cases of probability, we need to study various types of events.

2.3.1 TYPES OF EVENTS

Complementary events: Let E^c be the complementary event of E. Then we can say that E^c is the event that has all the outcomes that are not present in E. Also, $P(E \cup E^c) = P(S)$ or say $P(E^C) = 1 - P(E)$

Equally likely events: These are events in which the probability of happening of both events is equal. Let E1 and E2 be two events. Then they are called equally likely if $P(E1) = P(E2)$.

Mutually exclusive events: These are events which cannot occur together. Two events are said to be mutually exclusive if their intersection is zero. Let A and B be two events. Then they are mutually exclusive if $P(A \cap B) = 0$.

Collectively exhaustive events: These are events that collectively represent all the possible outcomes of a random experiment. Let C and D be two events of a random experiment. Then as collectively exhaustive events occur, $P(C \cup D) = P(S)$.

Independent events: Two events, A and B, are said to be independent if the occurrence or failure of A does not affect the occurrence or failure of B and vice versa. See Figure 2.1.

To understand the above types of events, let us take an example:

Solved Example 2.2: A bag containing marbles of three colours: three yellow, five brown and eight pink. Suppose a person draws one marble at a time and notes its colour and puts it back into the bag. He repeats this process several times. Let us define a few events that he may encounter in this experiment.

Event A: He draws a yellow marble.
Event B: He doesn't draw a yellow marble.
Event C: He draws a marble that is yellow or brown.
Event D: He draws a marble that is pink.
Event E: He draws a brown marble on the second draw.

Solution:
Event A: Probability of drawing a yellow marble = 3/16
Event B: Probability of drawing marble that is not yellow = (16 − 3)/16 = 13/16
Event C: Probability of drawing a yellow or brown marble = (3 + 5)/16 = 8/16
Event D: Probability of drawing a pink marble = 8/16
Event E: Probability of drawing a brown marble on the second draw = 5/16
    Event A and Event B are complementary events as P(A) + P(B) = 3/16 + 13/16 = 1
    Event C and Event D are equally likely events as P(C) = P(D)
    Event A and Event D are mutually exclusive events as $P(A \cap D) = 0$
    Event C and Event D are collectively exhaustive events as $P(C \cup D) = P(S) = 1$

Event D and Event E are independent events as the occurrence of event D doesn't affect the probability of happening of event E. After understanding the various types

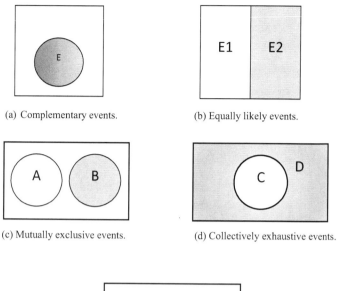

(a) Complementary events.   (b) Equally likely events.

(c) Mutually exclusive events.   (d) Collectively exhaustive events.

(e) Independent events.

FIGURE 2.1   Venn diagram representation of various types of events.

of events, now let us move back to the conditional probability, its definition, representation and applications.

Conditional probability is the probability calculated for two consecutive non-independent events. It can also be defined as the probability of happening of an event when the result of a previous event is known to us. It is denoted by P(B|A) = Probability of B when A has already happened. It can be formulated as:

$$P(B \mid A)\frac{P(A \, and \, B)}{P(A)} = \frac{P(A \cap B)}{P(A)}\cdots \tag{2.2}$$

2.4 BAYES THEOREM

This theorem is named after the British mathematician Thomas Bayes (eighteenth century). It is of great importance and is the application of conditional probability. This theorem allows us to update the probability calculated for a certain event to happen by incorporating additional details. To understand the Bayes theorem, let us consider an example:

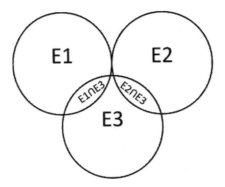

FIGURE 2.2   Bayes theorem.

Let us take two events to be mutually exclusive and whose outcomes are known, and one event whose outcome is not known. The probability of event 1(E1) and event 2(E1) to happen is 0.4 and 0.6 respectively. The probability of event 3(E3) to happen when E1 has already happened is 0.1, and the probability of E3 to happen when E2 has already happened is 0.3. Suppose it is given that E3 has happened. Then we need to determine the probability of E3 happening through E1.

These kinds of questions can be solved using Bayes theorem through the formula:

$$P(E1|E3) = \frac{P(E3|E1)}{P(E1|E3) + P(E2|E3)} \cdots$$

$$= \frac{P(E1)*P(E3|E1)}{[P(E1)*P(E3|E1)] + [P(E2)*P(E3|E2)]} \tag{2.3}$$

See Figure 2.2.

Solved Example 2.3: In the admission process of a school, the students applying for admission are shortlisted on the basis of a merit list and 30% of the students who apply get the chance for admission and the remaining students get a chance from a spot round after the merit list-based admission gets finished. If a student gets shortlisted in the merit list-based admission, then the chance of that student gaining admission is 50%. If a student on the wait list gets a chance to obtain admission through a spot round, he has an 80% chance of admission.

It the student receives admission to the school, what is the probability that he has gotten admission on the basis of the merit list?

Solution: Let the event of getting shortlisted through the merit list be E1
Event of getting a chance in a spot round is E2
And getting admission to the school is event E3

$$\text{Then, } P(E1) = 0.3 \quad P(E2) = 0.7$$

$$P(E3|E1) = 0.5 \quad P(E3|E2) = 0.8$$

We have to find a case when it is given that the student has received admission. Then the probability that he has gotten admission through the merit list is P(E1|E3):

$$P(E1 \mid E3) = \frac{P(E3 \mid E1)}{P(E3)} = \frac{P(E3 \mid E1)}{P(E3 \mid E1) + P(E3 \mid E2)}$$

$$= \frac{P(E1) * P(E3|E1)}{P(E1) * P(E3|E1) + P(E2) * P(E3|E2)} = \frac{0.3 * 0.5}{(0.3 * 0.5) + (0.7 * 0.8)}$$

$$= \frac{0.15}{0.15 + 0.56} = \frac{0.15}{0.71} = \mathbf{0.2112}$$

2.5   RANDOM VARIABLE

A random variable represents a function lying in the domain of a sample space of any random experiment and has a range of some set of real numbers. It is denoted by X(s). In probability theory and statistics, it is used to express the number of outcomes of an experiment. It has a distribution representing the likelihood of any occurring value of the possible outcome. Generally, a random variable is classified into three categories.

1. Discrete random variable (DRV)
2. Continuous random variable (CRV)
3. Mixed random variable (MRV)

DRV: A random variable X is called a discrete random variable if it can take only a countable number of values. In digital signal processing, this is a widely used tool to analyse a signal.

CRV: A random variable X is called a continuous random variable if it can take any value within one or more intervals.

MRV: A random variable X is called a mixed random variable if it has both types of values, some continuous and some discrete, or a random variable, which is neither purely continuous nor discrete.

2.6   DISTRIBUTION FUNCTIONS

Probability of a random variable can be represented in the form of a distribution function or a probability density function. This distribution describes all the possible values belonging to a particular range which a random variable can take. There are different types of distribution functions used to study random phenomena in different areas of applications which are based on prediction and multiple possibilities such as stock market prediction, sales growth, noise in a communication channel, weather forecast, results of any survey report and so on. Some popular distribution functions are discussed below.

2.6.1 BINOMIAL DISTRIBUTION

Binomial distribution simply tells us about the probability of success or failure of the event when an experiment is performed multiple times or repeated for n number of trials. This is another very popular type of discrete distribution used to analyse statistical data. A distribution is said to be binomial in nature when these four criteria are fulfilled:

1. Every time a trial is performed, the outcome must be either success or failure.
2. The number of observations must be a fixed number.
3. Every observation or outcome must be independent.
4. For each observation, the probability of success or failure must be equally likely.

Probability density function of a binomially distributed random variable is given as:

$$F(x) = \sum_{m=0}^{n} \left({}^{n}Cm \right).p^{m}q^{n-m}.\delta(x-m)... \tag{2.4}$$

To understand this more clearly, let us take an example of tossing a fair coin. This experiment will have only two possible outcomes, either heads or tails. Now let the falling of heads be a success and the falling of tails correspond to failure. Let p denotes the probability of success and q denote the probability of failure. When this experiment is repeated n times and we get m number of successes, then the number of failures will be n-m. The probability of getting m heads and n-m tails in an independent trial or event is given by:

$$P = p^{m}.q^{n-m}... \tag{2.5}$$

So, for n-trials the probability of getting m number of successes in any order is given by:

$$P(x = m) = P(m) = \left({}^{n}Cm \right).p^{m}q^{n-m}..., \tag{2.6}$$

where (m=0,1,2......n).

This type of distribution is called binomial distribution of order "n" and parameter "p." This serves as the basis function for the binomial test, which is very popular for statistical significance analysis. It is used to study and analyse the errors in digital communication systems and signal processing.

2.6.2 POISSON DISTRIBUTION

Poisson distribution is a special case of binomial distribution. When infinite trials of an experiment are performed with very little probability of success (infinitely small) such that the number of trials (n) approaches ∞ and the probability of success (p) approaches zero, but the product of both n and p is a constant value which is called the constant mean, rate denoted by λ, then it becomes a limiting case of binomial distribution. which is specifically called Poisson distribution. This distribution usually finds its application where a large number of events occur in a fixed time duration and each event is a rare case. Examples would be the number of accident cases arriving in a hospital between 1 and 3 p.m., the number of calls made in a specific time, and large data transmission in a communication system with a very low error rate. The probability density function of Poisson distribution is given by:

$$F(x) = \sum_{m=0}^{n} \frac{(e^{-\lambda}.\lambda^m)}{m!} . \delta(x - m)... \tag{2.7}$$

It becomes a limiting case of binomial distribution, provided that $np = \lambda$, so we can write,

$$Poisson\ distribution\ =\ \lim_{n \to \infty} Binomial\ distribution... \tag{2.8}$$

2.6.3 NORMAL DISTRIBUTION

This is also called Gaussian distribution. In general, maximum phenomena which are occurring naturally follow a normal distribution. These phenomena can be characterized by a random variable X and are distributed according to the probability density function given as:

$$F(x) = \frac{1}{\sqrt{2\pi\sigma^2}} . e^{-(x-m)^2/2\sigma^2} ..., \tag{2.9}$$

where
"m" stands for the mean of variable X and "σ" stands for variance.

A Gaussian distribution function is graphically represented by a bell-shaped curve which has its peak at the mean position, that is, at $x = m$. This curve is symmetric about its mean value. The area enclosed by this bell-shaped curve always equals one as the sum of all the probabilities of all possible outcomes of an event cannot exceed one. When the average value of normal distribution function is zero and the value of variance is equal to one, then it forms a special case, which is termed standard normal distribution. The typical normal distribution curve is shown in Figure 2.3.

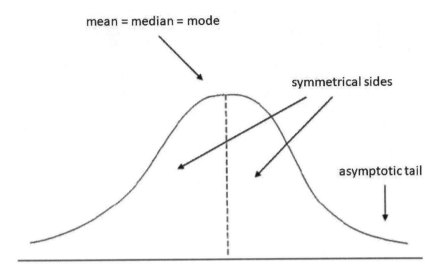

mean = median = mode

symmetrical sides

asymptotic tail

FIGURE 2.3   Normal distribution bell curve.

2.7   ESTIMATION

Estimation is basically a method to find the approximate value or the result of any experiment using the available data and information. Estimation is a part of statistics which is very useful in dealing with data science, finance and analysis problems in the field of signal processing. A rough estimation is made to determine whether the outcome or result will be in the desired range or not by observing the parameters involved. Sometimes the available information may be incomplete or uncertain, and on the basis of these parameters a guess is made which is assumed to be the approximate result or outcome (near to the true value). For example, in daily life we make a rough estimate of the house budget, or after the completion of any competitive exam an estimated value of cut-off marks is predicted, and in signal processing an estimation is carried out to find and measure the true value of a signal or a function. A primary goal of making an estimate is to obtain a range of outcomes which are near to the true value of results. If the estimated value exceeds the actual value, then it is said to be overestimated, and if the estimated value falls short of the actual value, then it is said to be underestimated.

The process of making an estimate is done by sampling. From a large population, a small sample is taken, and then after performing calculations on this small number, the outcome is projected over the entire population. The reliability of this totally depends on how the sample is taken, so one has to be very conscious while choosing a sample. For example, a bag contains two balls; one is white and other is black in colour. If a ball is taken out at random, it may turn out to be white (indicated by X = 0) or black (X = 1). Suppose 40 trials of this experiment are made and the outcomes observed were 18 times the white and 22 times the black ball. Therefore, by observing this, one can make the interpretation that the probability of getting a black ball is slightly higher than getting a white ball, but they are likely to be nearly equal.

This type of approach for making an estimation is called *maximum likelihood estimation* (MLE). Now suppose we decrease the number of trials for this experiment and this time only five trials are performed, observing the outcomes as four times white and one time black. In this case our estimate using the MLE approach will give a very unreliable result. This shows that as the sample size increases, the reliability of MLE approach also increases. For training large datasets, this approach is a good choice, but for a very small dataset, this approach could be a disaster. Therefore, to overcome this drawback, another approach is used which is called *maximum posteriori probability*. In this approach, assumptions based on prior knowledge about the outcomes are also taken into consideration along with the sample data. These two approaches are mainly incorporated into almost all machine learning algorithms for a probabilistic model and training datasets such as linear regression, Bayesian network design and neural network design.

2.8   STANDARD ERROR

This is the standard deviation of data or sampling distribution. The standard deviation is not exact but an estimation. It is denoted by "σ." If there are multiple sets of samples having multiple means, then the standard error is called the standard error of mean (SEM).

It is calculated by taking repeated samples and recording their means. This sample forms a set of different means, which has its own mean and variance. So in general, the standard error of mean gives us the measure of the dispersion of sample means around the population mean. Mathematically, it is represented as:

$$SE = \frac{\sigma}{\sqrt{n}}...,$$
(2.10)

where SE = standard error of the sample, σ = sample standard deviation, and n = number of samples

2.9   PROBABILITY OF ERROR

In any statistical modelling, an error can be considered a random variable which has a distributed probability over the entire range, and this distribution can be used to calculate the probability of error. It can be seen as the whole probability of the total error occurring in any prediction model, though it is not the sum of the individual probability of error of each predicted value. In statistical modelling, where predictions are made, the probability of error plays an important role. For example, in the linear regression model, and curve fitting, the difference between the predicted value and the true value is considered an error and for multiple values, probabilities of error are calculated, which can be helpful for determining the performance of the machine learning model. In hypothesis testing, the probability of error can be distinguished according to the type of error:

Type 1 error: in this case the probability of error is denoted by "α," and can be formulated as: $\alpha = 1 - specificity$

Type 2 error: in this case the probability of error is denoted by "β," and can be formulated as: $\beta = 1 = sensitivity$

LEARNING OUTCOMES

After studying this chapter, the students will be able to:

- Use necessary probability concepts and functions in the analysis of medical signal processing and applications.

Exercise

Q1. In an experiment, a card is selected at random and checked. If it is a face card, it is taken out of the deck; if it is a number card, it is put it back in the deck. This process is repeated several times. Determine the following:

    a. The probability of getting a number card in the first draw.

    b. The probability of getting a king in the second selection when first selection is known to be a jack.

    c. The probability of getting a face card in the third draw if it is known that the first two draws are face cards.

Q2. A bag of marbles contains two black marbles, five brown marbles and eight white marbles. A marble is taken out at random (without replacing it) and its colour is noted. What is the probability of getting a black marble in the second draw if a black marble is taken out in the first draw?

Q3. In a class of 60 students, 35 are boys and 25 are girls. A test is conducted in which 25 boys and 18 girls pass. A student is selected at random and his/her result is known as that he/she passed the test. Determine:

    a. The probability that the passed student is a boy.

    b. The probability that the passed student is a girl.

Q4. A coin is tossed five times and its result is recorded. What is the probability of getting at least four heads.?

Q5. On a test having 15 multiple choice questions, with each question having four options (a,b,c,d), determine the probability of getting five questions correct just by guessing. (Hint: use binomial distribution)

Q6. If X is a normally distributed random variable with mean value 20 and standard deviation equals to 2, determine:

    a. $P(X < 30)$

    b. $P(X > 15)$

3 Medical Data Acquisition and Pre-processing

LEARNING OBJECTIVES

This chapter aims to cover:

- Medical data formats
- Data augmentation and generation
- Data labelling, data cleaning and data normalization

3.1 MEDICAL DATA FORMATS

Medical data can be collected in different ways and accordingly, medical data is available in different forms such as electroencephalograph (EEG), electrocardiograph (ECG) and so on. There are some pictorial forms of representations such as computed tomography (CT) scan, magnetic resonance imaging (MRI) and son on, and also in the form of numerical measurements (lab results). Medical data can be used for various diagnostic and clinical research purposes. There are various formats available in which these medical data can be recorded and stored. Examples of such data formats are explained in this section.

3.1.1 DATA FORMATS FOR MEDICAL IMAGES

Medical imaging is a technique used to capture and store images of various body parts that can be helpful for diagnostic and treatment purposes. There are various techniques used by radiologists for capturing an image of body parts, such MRI, CT, radiographs or X-rays, ultrasound, positron emission tomography (PET), fluoroscopy, thermography, endoscopy and so on [1]. The images captured from these techniques are stored in various image files in different data formats. Image files are one of the standard ways to store the medical information in a computer. A medical image may contain one or a group of images that highlight some volumetric information or anatomical information on some part of the body. The captured images are stored using different file formats which describes the organization of image data inside the image file. Generally, four major file formats are used for storing, handling and working with medical images, Analyze, Neuroimaging Informatics Technology Initiative (NIfTI),

DOI: 10.1201/9781003097808-3

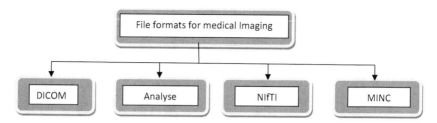

FIGURE 3.1   File formats for medical imaging.

MINC (Medical Imaging NetCDF), and Digital Imaging and Communications in Medicine (DICOM) [2], as shown in Figure 3.1. Brain tumour detection and treatment is the most emerging application of medical imaging techniques [3].

3.1.1.1   DICOM (Digital Imaging and Communications in Medicine)

This is the most commonly used file format for storing and transmitting biomedical images. This format enables the integration of biomedical imaging devices with printers, workstations, scanners servers and so on. The format is widely used in hospitals; DICOM files can be exchanged between two systems that are capable to receive data in DICOM format.

The DICOM file format includes the image file and the TCP/IP network communication protocol to communicate. There are numerous medical imaging modalities that utilize DICOM formats such as CT, MRI and PET. DICOM files can be viewed by using a variety of DICOM viewer software. Some software are 3Dim viewer, DICOM web viewer, Mango, Escape EMV and so on.

3.1.1.2   Analyse

Analyse is a software package which is used in the measuring and processing of multimodal images for biomedical applications. This format is also used in CT, MRI and PET for investigating various diseases of the body like cancer, tumours or any other abnormalities inside the different organs or parts of the body. The file stores the voxel-based volumes and the file format consist of two files; one is actual binary data with the extension '.img' and the other is a header file with the extension '.hdr' which keeps the information about voxel size and numbers.

3.1.1.3   NIfTI (Neuroimaging Informatics Technology Initiative)

This file format is most commonly used in neuroimaging and neuroradiology. It is an improved version of the Analyse file format. There are basically two file formats, NIfTI-1 and NIfTI-2. NIfTI-2 allows more data to be stored as compared to NIfTI-1.

3.1.1.4   MINC (Medical Imaging NetCDF)

MINC was built upon the NetCDF (Network Common Data Format) standard. MINC was designed to provide researchers the facility to store biomedical multimodal images with flexible and rich data support. There are several features of the MINC format, such as a header format to incorporate data acquisition and analysis history, a human readable self-documenting metadata to incorporate descriptive variables and attribute names, support for new modalities and platform independence [4].

3.1.2 MEDICAL DATA FORMATS FOR SIGNALS

Biomedical signals are recordings of various physiological activities like neural and cardiac rhythms that can be helpful for diagnostic and treatment purposes. Commonly used biomedical signals are EEG, ECG, electrooculogram (EOG), electromyogram (EMG) and so on, and these signals are generated by measuring the potential difference between the two electrodes. These recorded signals can be stored in various file formats as shown in Figure 3.2 [5].

3.1.2.1 EDF (European Data Format)

The EDF format is designed to incorporate multichannel data with different sampling rates. It includes data records and a header file. The header contains general (patient ID, start time etc.) and technical information (sampling rate, filtering, etc). Later development EDF+ allows discontinuous recordings, annotations and events in UTF-8 format. While EDF format is mostly used for polysomnography (PSG), EDF+ format finds its application in EEG, ECG, EMG and so on.

3.1.2.2 BDF (BioSemi Data Format)

This is the data format for BioSemi recording systems. The BDF file format is similar to the EDF format, the only difference being that the EDF file format doesn't support values other than int16, whereas the GDF (general data format) format supports int24 values and markers are stored as bitmasks, which is different from EDF+ [6].

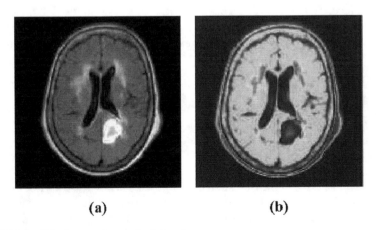

(a)   (b)

FIGURE 3.2   File formats for medical signals.

3.1.2.3 GDF (General Data Format)

This is used as a scientific medical data format which actually combines a number of features of various biomedical signals and creates a common file as a single file format. The GDF was introduced for addressing the drawbacks of the EDF. In the GDF format, an event table and a binary header are mainly included. The GDF was modified and the upgraded version of GDF was introduced in 2011 as GDF v2, which incorporates additional subject-specific information (gender, age, etc.), several standard codes for storing physical units and so on. The GDF file format can be applied to store various biomedical signals like EEG, ECG and so on [7].

3.2 DATA AUGMENTATION AND GENERATION

With the application of deep learning (DL) in the field of biomedical signal and image processing, there is a requirement for large datasets to get optimum results, but in collecting data in the biomedical field there are certain limitations which restrict the formation of larger datasets. The limitations can be in the form of a limited number of patients, physical impairments and unpleasant experiences for patients when data is recorded for longer durations. These limitations can be seen in various medical image modalities, such as EOG, EEG, EMG and ECG recordings and so on [8].

The problem of large datasets can be overcome by applying a technique called data augmentation. This technique involves the generation of a synthetic database from existing labelled samples, which helps the model learn the intra-class variations that can be observed. The key challenge is to generate the data while maintaining the correct label. Data augmentation helps improve the accuracy and stability of the deep learning models [9]. Based on data type (medical image or biomedical signal), the data augmentation technique is applied. The data augmentation for medical image data can be simply achieved by geometrical transformations like flipping, rotating, cropping, mirroring, adding noise and so on. However, for small datasets, the problem will not be resolved using this technique. So, another solution is generating entirely new synthetic images by using Generative adversarial networks (GAN). For bio-signals, a recently developed generative pre-trained transformer (GPT-2 and GPT-3) method created by Open AI is capable of generating synthetic signals such as EEG and EMG. The architecture and a detailed explanation of GAN can be found in [9, 10].

3.3 DATA LABELLING

Data labelling is an important part of data pre-processing when using machine learning, particularly in the case of supervised learning. It is the process of adding one or more relevant and informative labels (e.g. benign or malignant tumour in the case of biomedical images) to the raw data (text files, images. signals etc.) so that machine learning model can learn from it.

The machine learning classification technique falls into two categories, supervised and unsupervised learning. In the case of supervised learning, experts are required to label some data of the dataset, and then the supervised learning model passes this label information to the rest of the unlabelled data in the biomedical dataset. This helps the machine learning model make decisions correctly. In the case of unsupervised

TABLE 3.1
Feature Vectors x and Labels

Features	Labels
$X_1^{(1)}$ $X_1^{(2)}$ $X3^{(3)}$ ....$X_1^{(m)}$	y_1
$X_2^{(1)}$ $X_2^{(2)}$ $X2^{(3)}$ ....$X_2^{(m)}$	y_2
$X_3^{(1)}$ $X_3^{(2)}$ $X3^{(3)}$ ....$X_3^{(m)}$	y_3
....	..
....	..
$X_n^{(1)}$ $X_n^{(2)}$ $X_n^{(3)}$ ....$X_n^{(m)}$ y_n	y_n

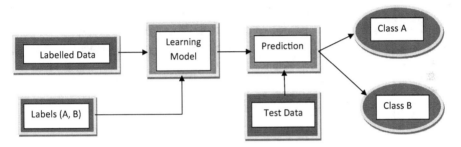

FIGURE 3.3　Labelling process for supervised learning model.

learning, labelling is not required as the learning model learns by itself and automatically partitions the data into two different datasets. In machine learning (ML) and deep learning (DL), the data used for learning must be labelled properly, which helps the machine learning model organize data properly and provide the desired results. The label should be discriminating, independent and informative. Signals can be labelled manually or by using algorithms. Labels can also be provided by using the signal labeller app in MATLAB [11].

Consider a dataset, as shown in Table 3.1, having feature vector X ranging from $X_1^{(1)}$ to $X_n^{(m)}$, where $X_1^{(1)}$ to $X_1^{(m)}$ are the same kind of feature and assigned the label y_1. Similarly, X_2, X_3 .... X_n represent different feature sets and are assigned labels from y_2 to y_n.

The importance of the labelling process for supervised learning can be explained with the help of the block diagram in Figure 3.3.

In the block diagram, the learning model is trained with the help of the labelled data and labels (e.g. A, B) as an input. After completion of the learning process, test data is applied to get classified into different classes.

3.4　DATA CLEANING

When using machine learning for data processing, it is highly recommended to use quality data for more accuracy. Medical data is used for diagnosis and other important applications, and thus it becomes necessary to make the data clean and proper so that the data can produce appropriate and complete results. There are some indicators of quality data, that is, accuracy, completeness, consistency, relevancy, validity and uniformity. Enhancing the data quality is necessary to resolve these issues. The quality of the data is considerably improved by data cleaning that involves the problem of repetitive object detection, missing data and outlier, thus minimizing the risk of wrong and inaccurate conclusions.

Earlier, the cleaning of medical data was done manually through conventional approaches aimed at checking abnormal and missing values, and the process involved used to be time-consuming, expensive and tedious. Moreover, the cleaning does not ensure that the results are suitable for medical applications with optimal performance. Therefore, there is a requirement to automate the process. One approach to the general cleaning process can be found in [12].

Mainly, three important steps are required in the medical data cleaning process, as follows: (1) identification of the data which is corrupted by some anomalies or impurities, (2) consideration of the corrupted data as missing data and (3) imputing the missing data [12].

There are several other cleaning approaches proposed by researchers to deal with the problem of corrupt data. The cleaning process can be divided into two categories: the statistical approach and the machine learning approach to handle missing data [13].

3.4.1 STATISTICAL APPROACH

In this approach, missing data can be handled by simply applying a statistical algorithm. There are several ways; some of them are explained in this section.

3.4.1.1 Listwise Deletion

This is the traditional approach in which the missing or corrupted data is simply omitted, and the data processing takes place with the remaining dataset. Listwise deletion is common approach in most of the data analysis process.

3.4.1.2 Pairwise Deletion

In this technique, missing data will not be deleted but can be used for analysis of other variables which are present. For example, if a data contains values for three variables: v1, v2 and v3, and suppose the values corresponding to v1 are missing, then complete data will not get deleted but the statistical analysis will continue with other variable values that are present in the corrupted data.

3.4.1.3 Multiple Imputation

The method discussed above suffers from noises due to imputation; therefore, to overcome this problem, multiple imputations are used. In this technique, missing values in a data can be imputed by a number of acceptable values which possess some uncertainty about the original values of the data. Therefore, this technique produces a number of data that correspond to a single data and after that, the average is taken to form a single data.

3.4.1.4   Maximum Likelihood Imputation

In this technique, imputation is done from the multivariate maximum likelihood function. This technique does not impute any data but calculates the maximum likelihood estimation from the complete observed data. This technique has the advantage that careful selection of a variable is not required as is done in previous methods.

However, statistical imputation techniques still suffer from a loss of information that leads to incorrect conclusions. Thus, machine learning methods become extremely important for efficient and correct imputation, which considers all values and uncertainty involved and A few important machine learning methods are briefly explained here.

3.4.2   Machine Learning for Data Imputation

The current literature suggests that the research on imputation using machine learning methods is very limited and those studies which are available, are not focused. Few studies suggest that machine learning can be of great importance in obtaining satisfactory imputation results.

This section discusses some of the data imputation methods using machine learning techniques [13].

3.4.2.1   K-Nearest Neighbour (KNN)

This method is reported as a simple and effective method that can be used for the imputation of missing data. In this technique, K-nearest neighbour is identified from the sample data available for a variable and then the missing data is imputed from the average values of KNN of non-missing data. The nearest neighbour is calculated on the basis of Euclidean distance.

3.4.2.2   Bayesian Network (BN)

The characteristic of BN is its ability to model the causal relationship between the variables and uncertainty, which makes it a prominent tool in various medical applications. The BN model contains a probabilistic relationship between the variables. BN is based on the graphical format, and the BN model requires each variable to be in the form of a node, and the causal relationship is represented by an arc and the conditional probabilities. The probability either can be in tabulated form or in the form of formulas. A properly designed BN provides the expected value of missing variables [14].

There are some other advanced techniques also mentioned by researchers like the co-appearance based analysis for incorrect records and attribute-values detection (CAIRAD) and the framework for imputing missing values using co-appearance, correlation and similarity analysis (FIMUS), which are discussed in this section. For detecting corrupt data, the CAIRAD [15] method is suggested that utilizes a co-appearance matrix for holding the number of co-occurrences of each attribute-value pair present in the dataset. The CAIRAD can provide a clean dataset effectively with the help of identification and removal of noisy records from the original dataset. An imputation of missing value can be done by using the technique FIMUS [16], which generalizes the numerical attribute values into a number of categories that assist in calculating the co-appearances of the data values as compared to other values having the other attributes.

3.5 DATA NORMALIZATION

It is very important that data being implemented lies in some specific ranges, and this task is done by data normalization. This is considered a technique that works by restricting the data values of all the variables within a predetermined range. Data normalization is a pre-processing technique that is basically employed before the feature selection and classification. The features that are generated by different feature extraction methods may have different dynamic ranges. Therefore, normalization techniques are used to equalize the ranges of the features to maintain computation similarity.

There are two categories of normalization techniques: linear and non-linear normalization. The linear normalization technique is used when the data is evenly distributed, and non-linear normalization is used when the data is not evenly distributed. There are various normalization techniques available. However, the selection of normalization

TABLE 3.2
Normalization Techniques and Formulas

S.no	Normalization Technique	Formula	Usage condition
1	Linear Scaling	$x' = (x - x_{min})/(x_{max} - x_{min})$	Uniformly distributed features across a fixed range. Squashes the data in the range [0,1]
2	Min-Max Scaling	$x' = (x - x_{min}) (\max X_{new} - \min X_{new}) + \min X_{new}$ $(x_{max} - x_{min})$	Linear normalization technique squashes the data in the range [max X_{new},min X_{new}]
3	Clipping	if x > max, then x' = max. if x < min, then x' = min	If some extreme outliers are present in the features.
4	Log Scaling	$x' = \log(x)$	If the power law is observed in features
5	Z-score	$x' = (x - \mu) / \sigma$ μ = mean, σ = standard deviation	If no extreme outliers are present in the features
6	Softmax scaling	$x' = 1/(1 + e^{-y})$ & $y = x_i - \mu /r\sigma$ r = user defined parameter, μ = mean, σ = standard deviation	Non-linear normalization technique, based on non-linear function, used when data is not evenly distributed, and limits the range [0,1]

technique is a very critical task, because applying an incorrect technique may cause changes in the data structure that may further affect the results and performance of machine learning models [17].

Different normalization techniques with formulas are presented in Table 3.2.

LEARNING OUTCOMES

After completion of this chapter, learners/students will be able to explain:

- Importance of medical data
- Challenges in medical data handling
- Data normalization and its importance
- Role of machine learning in data imputation

REFERENCES

1. Kasban, Hany, El-bendary, Mohsen, & Salama, Dina. (2015). A comparative study of medical imaging techniques. *International Journal of Information Science and Intelligent System, 4*, 37–58.
2. Larobina, M., & Murino, L. (2013). Medical image file formats. *Journal of Digital Imaging, 27*(2), 200–206. https://doi.org/10.1007/s10278-013-9657-9
3. Wu, M.-N., Lin, C.-C., & Chang, C.-C. (2007). Brain tumor detection using color-based k-means clustering segmentation, *Third International Conference on Intelligent Information Hiding and Multimedia Signal Processing* (IIH-MSP 2007). https//doi.org/10.1109/IIH-MSP.2007.356
4. Vincent et al. (2016). MINC 2.0: A flexible format for multi-modal images, *Frontiers in Neuroinformatics,* 10. https://doi.org/10.3389/fninf.2016.00035
5. Vidaurre, C., Sander, T. H., & Schlögl, A. (2011). BioSig: The free and open source software library for biomedical signal processing. *Computational Intelligence and Neuroscience, 2011*, 1–12. https://doi.org/10.1155/2011/935364
6. Schlögl, A. (2009). An overview on data formats for biomedical signals. In O. Dössel & W. C. Schlegel (Eds.), *Image Processing, Biosignal Processing, Modelling and Simulation, Biomechanics* (Vol. 25/IV, pp. 1557–1560). (IFMBE Proceedings). Springer.
7. General data format for biomedical signals. (2018, June 14). In *Wikipedia*. https://en.wikipedia.org/w/index.php?title=General_Data_Format_for_Biomedical_Signals&oldid=845882409.
8 Tsinganos, P., Cornelis, B., Cornelis, J., Jansen, B., & Skodras, A. (2020). Data augmentation of surface electromyography for hand gesture recognition. *Sensors, 20*(17), 4892. https://doi.org/10.3390/s20174892
9. Lashgari, E., Liang, D., & Maoz, U. (2020). Data augmentation for deep-learning-based electroencephalography. *Journal of Neuroscience Methods, 346*, 108885. https://doi.org/10.1016/j.jneumeth.2020.108885
10. Haradal, Shota, Hayashi, Hideaki, & Uchida, Seiichi. (2018). Biosignal data augmentation based on generative adversarial networks. *2018 Annual International Conference of the IEEE Engineering in Medicine and Biology Society* (EMBC), 2018, pp. 368–371. https://doi.org/10.1109/EMBC.2018.8512396
11. Hsun-Hsien, Chang, & Jose, M. F. Moura (2009). Biomedical signal processing. In Myer Kutz (Ed.), *Biomedical Engineering and Design Handbook* (Vol. 1, ch. 22).

McGraw   Hill.   www.accessengineeringlibrary.com/content/book/9780071498388/chapter/chapter22

12. Koren, A., Jurčević, M., & Prasad, R. (2020). Comparison of data-driven models for cleaning eHealth sensor data: Use case on ECG signal. *Wireless Personal Communications, 114*(2), 1501–1517. https://doi.org/10.1007/s11277-020-07435-7

13. Abidin, N. Z., Ismail, A. R., & Emran, N. (2018). Performance analysis of machine learning algorithms for missing value imputation. *International Journal of Advanced Computer Science and Applications, 9*(6), 442–447. https://doi.org/10.14569/ijacsa.2018.090660

14. Huei et al. (2008). Exploiting missing clinical data in Bayesian network modeling for predicting medical problems. *Journal of Biomedical Informatics, 41*(1), 1–14, https://doi.org/10.1016/j.jbi.2007.06.001.

15. Rahman, M. G., Islam, M. Z., Bossomaier, T., & Gao, J. (2012). CAIRAD: A co-appearance-based analysis for incorrect records and attribute-values detection. *The 2012 International Joint Conference on Neural Networks (IJCNN)*, 2012, pp. 1–10. https://doi.org/10.1109/IJCNN.2012.6252669.

16. Rahman, M. G., & Islam, M. Z. (2014). FIMUS: A framework for imputing missing values using co-appearance, correlation and similarity analysis. *Knowledge-Based Systems, 56*, 311–327. https://doi.org/10.1016/j.knosys.2013.12.005

17. Kumar Singh, B., Verma, K., & S. Thoke, A. (2015). Investigations on impact of feature normalization techniques on classifier's performance in breast tumor classification. *International Journal of Computer Applications, 116*(19), 11–15. https://doi.org/10.5120/20443-2793

4 Medical Image Processing

DOI: 10.1201/9781003097808-4

LEARNING OBJECTIVES

This chapter aims to cover:

- Importance of image processing in medical field
- Different imaging modalities with their applications, advantages and limitations
- Medical image enhancement and de-noising
- Medical image segmentation

The significant improvement in the quality of medical care for patients is witnessed with the introduction of advanced imaging techniques. Accuracy and precision in clinical practices as well as the development of equipment are necessary for the medical field [1]. Medical imaging is playing a vital role in the health sector as it aims to reduce the cost and early detection of disease [2]. Some application areas of imaging technologies include surgery, nuclear medicine, diagnosis in the field of radiology and so on.

4.1 MEDICAL IMAGE MODALITIES, THEIR APPLICATIONS, ADVANTAGES AND LIMITATIONS

In the modern healthcare system, the use of a computer-aided diagnosis (CAD) system is used that employs computer algorithms to achieve better analysis and effective diagnosis processes of various types of medical images. The CAD acquires medical images for a particular disease and applies various types of methods aimed at enhancement, segmentation and analysis of the images. Various types of medical images are captured for different types of diseases, such as computed tomography (CT), X-ray, mammography, radiographs, magnetic resonance imaging (MRI) and so on. A rapid growth in technology has made the acquisition of internal structures a commonplace in three (3D) and four-dimensional (4D) representations. Some of the available imaging modalities used in the medical field are discussed next.

4.1.1 RADIOGRAPHY

Radiography is an imaging technique that uses X-rays or some ionizing and non-ionizing radiation for diagnostic procedures to view the internal parts of the body. An image receptor is used to highlight the differences in tissue densities employing attenuation, or in the case of ionizing radiation, the absorption of X-ray photons by the denser substances. Fluoroscopy and projectional radiography are two forms of radiography.

Although 3D technologies have shown advancement in the field of radiography, the 2D technologies still find their application due to their low cost, good resolution and low radiation.

- *Projectional radiography:* This method makes use of the exposure of an object to X-rays or other forms of electromagnetic radiation and hence captures the shadow. Projectional radiography offers a low cost and a high diagnostic yield.
- *Fluoroscopy:* Fluoroscopy was invented by Thomas Edison and this technique is mainly performed to view the movement of any contrast agent along with a tissue, or as a guide in the case of angioplasty, pacemaker insertion, and so on [2]. In these types of medical image modalities, interior parts of the human body are detected using real-time images. These can be produced using images such as X-rays or radiographs. Further, an image receptor is used to convert the radiation into an image which passes through the affected part.

4.1.2 NUCLEAR MEDICINE

Radioactive materials are used in this modality of medical imaging and the diagnosis is carried out by using a radiograph employing the radioactive technology of imaging. The different structures of organs can be easily highlighted using this method [2]. This modality is a combination of disciplines, including chemistry, computer technology, medicine and many others. Nuclear imaging enables us to view the structure of organs and tissue as well as their function. Some techniques available for diagnostic nuclear medicine are comprised of two main types, positron emission tomography (PET) and single photon emission computed tomography (SPECT).

4.1.2.1 Positron Emission Tomography (PET)

This modality of imaging uses radioactive substances, also known as radiotracers, for visualizing and measuring the changes in metabolic processes, depending on the target process inside the body. A pharmaceutical is injected into the body and gamma rays are emitted and detected by cameras to form a 3D image. The reconstruction of PET scan images can be done using a CT scan. High initial as well as ongoing operating costs are the limitations of a PET scanner.

4.1.3 ELASTOGRAPHY

This is a medical imaging modality that maps the elastic property and stiffness of soft tissue. The presence of a disease is diagnosed depending on whether the tissue is soft or hard [2]. It can further be used to carry out additional diagnostic information such as to guide biopsies or to replace them entirely as the former is completely non-invasive. Magnetic resonance elastography (MRE), ultrasound elastography and optical coherence tomography are the various types of elastography techniques being used. Some of the ultrasound elastographic techniques are acoustic radiation force impulse imaging (ARFI), shear-wave elasticity imaging (SWEI), supersonic shear imaging (SSI) and transient elastography.

4.1.4 PHOTOACOUSTIC IMAGING

The photoacoustic effect is used in this technique of medical imaging in which the non-ionizing laser pulses transfer energy to body tissues, and the energy is absorbed and converted into heat, which causes a thermoelastic expansion. Ultrasound waves are generated by this expansion and detected by the transducer, which creates images of optical absorption contrast in tissues. The two types of photoacoustic imaging systems are photoacoustic tomography (PAT) (also known as thermos-acoustic computed tomography (TAT)) and photoacoustic microscopy (PAM).

4.1.5 TOMOGRAPHY

Tomography is an imaging technique in which the X-ray images of deep internal parts are obtained by focusing on a specific plane inside the body [2]. These images are obtained depending upon a mathematical tomographic reconstruction algorithm, which is produced from multiple projection radiographs. Single photon emission computed tomography (SPECT) from gamma rays, CT from X-ray, PET from positron emission and so on are some types of tomography techniques.

- *X-ray Computed Tomography (CT)*

This technique refers to a computerized X-ray imaging modality. In this modality, a narrow X-ray beam is pointed at the patient and is rotated around the body. The signals thus produced are processed by the computer, which generates cross-sectional images. Using mathematical techniques, CT constructs a 2D image slice of the patient, which can either be displayed individually or stacked together to generate a 3D image of the patient. This method has the advantage of being able to rotate the 3D image or to view slices in succession, so as to find the location of the problem.

4.1.6 MAGNETIC RESONANCE IMAGING (MRI)

Magnetic resonance imaging (MRI) is a medical imaging technique that implements a strong magnetic field and radio waves for the generation of organs and tissues images. MRI does not involve X-rays or any ionizing radiation, unlike CT and PET scans [2]. The radio waves re-align the hydrogen atoms which exist normally inside the body without causing any kind of chemical changes within the tissues. The hydrogen atoms emit different amounts of energy, which depend upon the type of tissue. This energy is further captured by the scanner which gathers this information. A computer processes this information to create a series of images showing thin slices of the body, which can be read by the radiologist at different angles. MRI finds its applications to image knee and shoulder injuries, breast cancer screening for women who are at high risk of breast cancer tumours, diseases related to liver and other abdominal organs, and many other areas.

4.1.7 ULTRASOUND IMAGING TECHNIQUES

Ultrasound imaging is one of the most commonly used medical imaging modalities in the areas of cardiology, obstetrics, gynaecology and so on [3]. Ultrasound imaging techniques utilize the involvement of sound waves with living tissue to form an image. Medical ultrasound is categorized into two types: diagnostic and therapeutic. *Diagnostic ultrasound* is a non-invasive method used for the imaging of the inside of the body. In this case, the transducer of the ultrasound probe produces sound waves whose frequencies are above 20 KHz, and in some transducers very high frequency in the range of megahertz (MHz) is also produced. The ultrasound, which is used in the diagnostic process, also known as diagnostic ultrasound, can be classified into two main types namely functional and anatomical ultrasound. The images of internal organs or other structures of the human body are created by the anatomical ultrasound technique; whereas movement and velocity of tissue or blood are recorded in functional ultrasound, which is also used to collect the physical characteristics, hardness and softness of the tissues. The technique most frequently used for treatment of chronic pain and healing of tissues is *therapeutic ultrasound*. This employs sound waves which are above range of human hearing.

Figure 4.1 shows a basic block diagram of an ultrasound imaging system. The principal components of a basic ultrasound imaging system include a central processing unit (CPU), a transducer probe, a monitor, a keyboard, disk storage devices

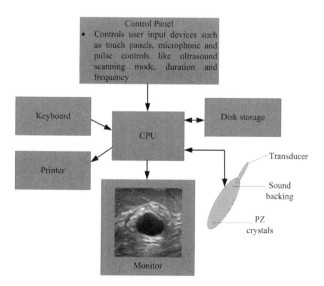

FIGURE 4.1   A typical block diagram of an ultrasound imaging system.

and a printer. The most vital component is the transducer probe. It generates the sound waves and also receives the reflected echoes using the phenomenon of the piezoelectric effect. The piezoelectric crystals within the transducer vibrate when they are exposed to small electrical currents, and hence produce sound waves. These sound waves are focused on a beam and thus transmitted through the soft tissues of the body and target organ. Each tissue has slightly different acoustic impedance, which depends upon the tissue density. Some sound waves which are reflected due to the mismatch of acoustic impedance produce a small current by interaction with the piezoelectric crystals in the transducer. The CPU controls and processes the input to the other components like the transducer and monitor, and the image thus constructed is displayed on a monitor, stored on a disk or printed.

4.2 MEDICAL IMAGE ENHANCEMENT

Acquired images may not always provide the quality needed for the desired analysis. Even for medical images, say, with acceptable quality, certain regions, features or components often need to be emphasized and highlighted. This may help physicians make a better diagnosis [4]. If the quality of images is not proper, then the medical diagnosis and analysis will be adversely affected and thus a suitable method of image de-noising or image enhancement is necessary.

Image enhancement techniques are regarded as computational algorithms that receive and process an image to generate an image of better quality that can be subjected to the application so that better understanding and interpretation of the image can be made in the application and we can get proper output. The enhancement aims at achieving either better image quality or enhanced visual appearance, and accordingly the methods are suggested for improving the images for specific applications. Image quality improvement or visual appearance improvement can be achieved by manipulating the greyscale values of the pixels directly, modifying its attributes or modifying the Fourier contents, and make it more suitable for a given task. Figure 4.2 shows the different image enhancement methods. Based on the two main objectives of image enhancement, the methods can broadly be categorized into two types:

- *Spatial Domain Techniques: Histogram equalization, masking, point processing, logarithmic operation and so on.*
- *Frequency Domain Techniques: Fourier transform-based image enhancement method*

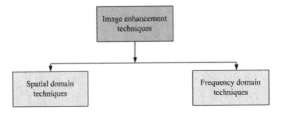

FIGURE 4.2 Classification of image enhancement methods.

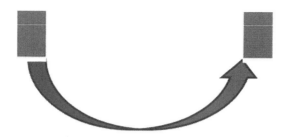

FIGURE 4.3   Point processing of image enhancement.

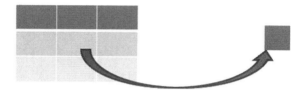

FIGURE 4.4   Masking operation.

Classification of Enhancement Techniques in Space Domain: In this method, we directly modify the pixel attributes such as greyscale values, colour, texture and so on. There are a number of methods available for spatial image enhancement, and a few of them are histogram modification, contrast enhancement, point processing, masking operation and so on. One such method is shown in Figure 4.3 for point processing, in which the pixel manipulation is being performed point-wise, choosing a pixel and performing the modification.

We can also use a mask of a suitable dimension in the spatial domain and apply it over the image to improve the quality, such as contrast improvement, brightness correction and so on. Figure 4.4 shows how this operation can be performed on an image. The mask chosen can slide over the input image from the left to the right corner in a top-to-bottom approach until all pixels of the image are covered.

The image negative or complement method plays an important role in several applications such as cancer detection. One such example is shown in Figure 4.5. In this figure, a mammogram, which is used in breast cancer diagnosis, is complemented and its negative prominently shows tissue structure [5].

Logarithmic transformation can be used as non-linear transformation of greyscale values employing a characteristic shown in Figure 4.6. The greyscale values will be modified as per the input-output characteristic illustrated in the diagram. There may be many similar power law transforms which can be applied over the input image, and the range of greyscale values can be extended or altered according to the non-linear transformation function.

Contrast is an important attribute in medical imaging and its value can be corrected in both the domains of enhancement. An example of contrast enhancement can be seen in Figure 4.7. This is especially helpful in highlighting the cancerous tissues visible in mammograms during breast cancer detection and diagnosis [6].

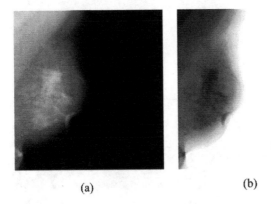

(a)   (b)

FIGURE 4.5   Image complement of a mammogram (a) Original image (b) Complement image.

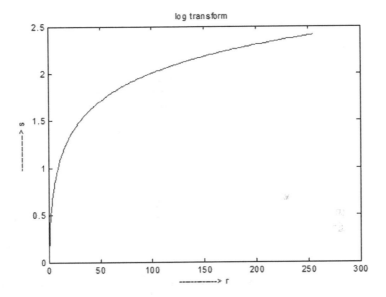

FIGURE 4.6   Logarithmic transformation.

4.3   BASICS OF HISTOGRAM

Histogram is a term that appears frequently in the discussion of image enhancement both in the spatial and the frequency domain, and thus we discuss some necessary basics of histogram in this section. The histogram of a digital image with grey levels in the range of $[0, L-1]$ is a discrete function $h(r_k) = n_k$, where r_k is the kth grey level and n_k is the number of pixels in the image having grey-level r_k. Figure 4.8 shows a typical histogram and histograms of a few images. The intensity distribution and corresponding number of pixels are plotted in the histogram, which helps in choosing a suitable range of values that we want to modify in the enhancement process. We

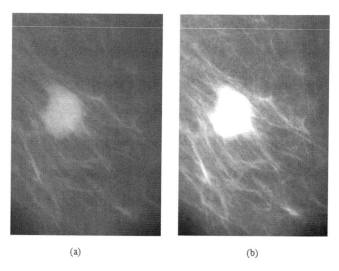

(a)   (b)

FIGURE 4.7   Contrast enhancement ((a) Original image (b) image with enhanced contrast).

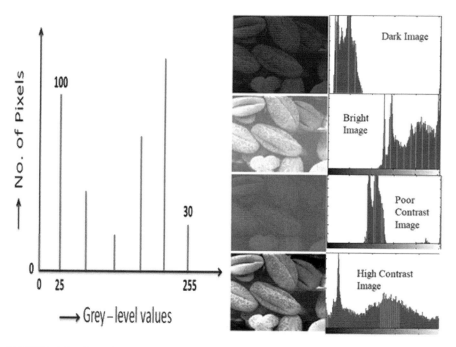

FIGURE 4.8   A typical histogram and histograms of images having different values of contrast.

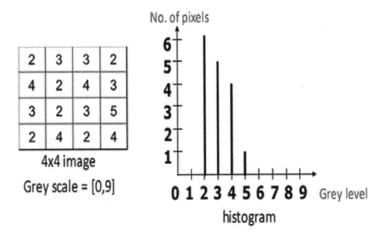

No. of pixels

FIGURE 4.9 Histogram of input image.

can clearly see that the bright image has a larger number of pixels in a higher grey-scale value range, whereas for the dark image, the pixels are aligned towards lower intensity values.

Properties of the image histogram that can be seen in Figure 4.8, are:

- Histogram clustered at low end: Dark Image
- Histogram clustered at high end: Bright Image
- Histogram with a small spread: Low-contrast Image
- Histogram with a wide spread: High-contrast Image

A normalized histogram is given by $p(r\_k) = n\_k/n$ for $k = 0,1, ...\ L - 1$ and n is the total number of pixels in the image. That is, $p(r\_k)$ gives an estimate of the probability of occurrence of grey-level r_k.

Histogram Equalization: A technique where the histogram of the resultant image is as flat as possible. The theoretical basis for histogram evaluation involves probability theory, where we treat the histogram as the probability distribution of the grey levels. Its function is similar to that of a histogram stretched image, but often provides more visually pleasing results across a wider range of images. In Figure 4.9, we can see a histogram of a representative image (shown in the first part of the figure as a matrix) and its histogram. A histogram after equalization with modified greyscale values in the image (matrix) can be seen in Figure 4.10. Figure 4.11 shows an example of histogram equalization where a mammogram is enhanced by using the equalization approach.

As discussed, and highlighted with the help of the examples above, we can understand that the direct manipulation of pixels' values is done through spatial domain methods, and we obtain an enhanced or better image. In the transom domain, we modify the transform of the image and later we get the inverse transform of the image,

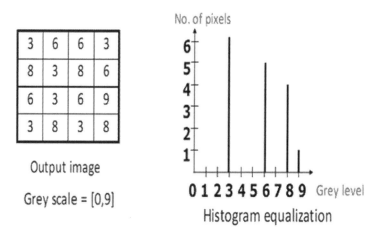

FIGURE 4.10 Histogram of output image after histogram equalization.

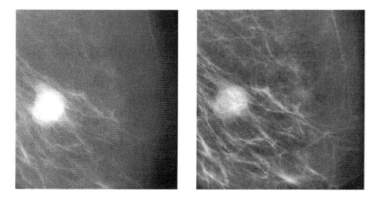

FIGURE 4.11 An example of histogram equalization.

subjecting it to an appropriate filtering. In spatial domain processing, the operation is performed on the pixels using the mathematical formula in Equation (4.1),

$$g(x, y) = T[f(x, y)]. \tag{4.1}$$

Here, $f(x, y)$ is the input image, $g(x, y)$ is the output enhanced image, and T denotes the operator defined on f applied over neighbouring pixels (x,y).

T can be defined in its simplest form when the size of the neighbourhood is 1×1, which means a single pixel. In this case, T resembles a grey-level transformation function given by:

$$s = T(r), \tag{4.2}$$

where r and s represent the grey levels of f(x,y) and g(x,y) at any point (x,y).

These techniques are known as *point processing* techniques, as the enhancement at any point depends only upon the grey level at that point. Another approach is *mask processing*, in which the larger neighbourhood allows more flexibility. It makes use of *masks* for this approach. The three commonly used functions for image enhancement are explained here.

- *Image Negatives:* The negative transformation is used to obtain the negative of an image whose grey levels lie in the range [0, L − 1]. It is denoted by the following expression:

$$s = L - 1 - r. \tag{4.3}$$

- *Log Transformations:* The log transformation is commonly expressed as:

$$s = c \log(1 + r), \tag{4.4}$$

where c is a constant and $r \geq 0$.

- *Power-law Transformations:* The basic representation of a power-law transformation is:

$$s = cr^{\gamma}. \tag{4.5}$$

Contrast stretching, grey-level slicing, bit-plane slicing, and histogram equalization are some of the other commonly used techniques for image enhancement in the spatial domain [7].

In frequency domain processing, the Fourier transform of the image (FT_1) is calculated as shown in Figure 4.12. After this, all the enhancement operations are carried out and the inverse Fourier transform is performed on the FT_1 image to obtain the desired image [8]. The purpose of these enhancement operations is to modify the

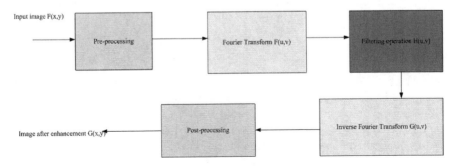

FIGURE 4.12 Frequency domain operations.

brightness, contrast or grey levels of the image. By making use of this method, we can improve the quality of an image by making changes in its transform coefficient functions. Low-pass filters, high-pass filters and homomorphic filtering are the basic types of filter methods used in frequency domain processing. The advantages of frequency domain processing are its low complexity for computations. The major drawback of this method is that it cannot enhance all parts of the image and focuses on particular parts only. This means it does not produce a clear picture of the background.

4.4   MEDICAL IMAGE DE-NOISING

The removal of various types of noise from an image is a vital step in image processing [9]. Noise is inevitably introduced into medical images during the process of image storage, transmission and acquisition [10]. The noise degrades the image quality by blurring its boundaries and further suppressing its structural details, which makes it difficult for medical diagnosis. Thus, a good image de-noising model requires that it should completely remove the noise by preserving important image features.

Digital images play a vital role in the field of medical imaging such as ultrasound imaging, CT and MRI [11]. Image de-noising is an essential step when the acquired image is degraded in quality and needs to be restored [3]. Different types of noise are present in images acquired from different modalities. Image de-noising methods can be mainly categorized into two types, spatial filtering and transform domain filtering, as shown in Figure 4.13.

4.4.1   SPATIAL FILTERING

This is considered the traditional way to remove noise from the image [9]. Spatial filtering is the most commonly used form of filtering to remove additive noise [12].

It can further be classified into two different categories: linear filters and non-linear filters [11].

4.4.1.1   Linear Filters

There are several filters which work linearly and enhance images directly in the spatial domain directly. The most common noise, Gaussian noise, is filtered out by a linear filter such as a mean filter. Sharp contents such as edges, blurs and other similar minute details are filtered by linear filters. Mean and Wiener filters are popular examples of linear filtering methods.

- *Mean filter*

The smoothing operation is performed and intensity variations are reduced by the mean filter. The operation is performed over neighbourhood pixels, and abrupt variations are replaced by some mean values in this method. This is why the mean filter is also called an averaging filter, as it provides a masking operation by which the mean value replaces the neighbourhood pixels [11] [12]. The main disadvantage of this filter is that edge-preserving criteria are poor.

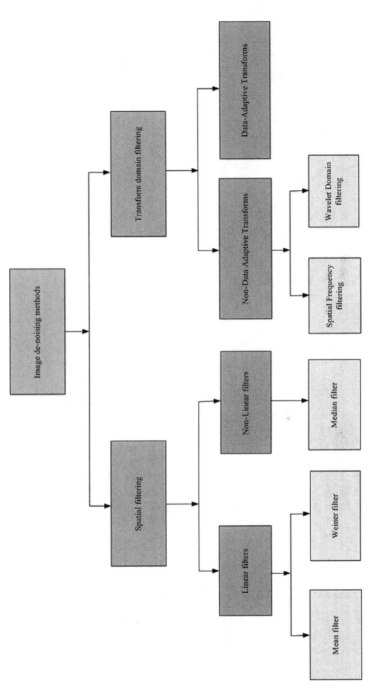

FIGURE 4.13 Various de-noising techniques used in medical image processing.

- *Wiener Filter*

Weiner filtering essentially needs knowledge about the spectra of the original signal and noise, and it gives good results only if the underlying signal is smooth [11]. The desired frequency response can be obtained using this filter.

4.4.1.2 Non-linear Filters

Non-linear filters find their applications when there is multiplicative kind of noise [9] [12]. This filter removes noise, but it causes the blurring of the images, which makes the edges invisible.

- *Median Filter*

Median filtering is carried out by obtaining the median value and then replacing each value in the window with the pixel's median value [9] [12] [13]. The median filter uses window size of 3×3, 5×5, or 7×7 [11]. Median filters are robust filters and used for providing smoothness in image-processing applications. The advantage of the median filter is that it is much less sensitive to outliers. Hence, it can remove them without degrading the sharpness of the image.

4.4.2 Transform Domain Filtering

Transform domain filtering is classified into two categories according to the choice of basic functions: non-data adaptive transform and data-adaptive transform [14].

4.4.2.1 Non-data Adaptive Transform

- *Spatial Frequency Filtering*

It implements low-pass filters using fast Fourier transform (FFT) [9]. A cut-off frequency is decided and the noise is removed by adapting a frequency-domain filter in which the components of noise are de-correlated from the useful signal. One disadvantage of FFT is that the information is lost and thus low-pass filtering results in the smearing of the edges.

- *Wavelet Domain Filtering*

The Wavelet domain is implemented usually because the discrete wavelet transform (DWT) of a noisy image has few coefficients with a high signal-to-noise ratio (SNR). Inverse DWT is used to reconstruct the image after the removal of coefficients with low SNR. Hence, the noise is removed or filtered. One advantage of wavelet-based methods is that they give both time and frequency localization.

4.4.2.2 Data-Adaptive Transforms

Non-Gaussian noise is reduced by a de-noising method using independent component analysis (ICA) and considered as a non-learning method of enhancement [9]. The salient feature of this method is that the noise is assumed as non-Gaussian and can enhance the signal content using both the distributions, Gaussian as well as non-Gaussian. The main drawback lies in the high computational cost involved in this method because the window sliding takes time for completing the operation over a sample data.

4.5 SEGMENTATION

Image segmentation is the process of partitioning an image into meaningful regions that are correlated to areas contained in the image [15]. The segmentation in medical image processing is of great importance as it divides the medical images into some distinct non-overlapping regions or partitions. Partitioning is applied using suitable criteria or constraints that may be some similarity or homogeneity metrics. The basic procedure consists of subdividing a particular image into various regions or parts. This process should stop when the objects of interest have been isolated. Figure 4.14 shows the various segmentation techniques used in image processing.

The image segmentation techniques are categorized as:

(i) Discontinuity-based and (ii) Similarity-based techniques.

The segmentation methods that follow the discontinuity property of pixels fall under the boundary or edges-based techniques [7]. The three common types of grey-level discontinuities are points, lines and edges. Similarity-based techniques are based on grouping the pixels in the image based on a certain similar attribute like colour, intensity and so on. In thresholding, a greyscale or colour image is converted to a binary image depending upon a threshold value. The image is partitioned into regions by considering the boundaries between regions corresponding to discontinuities in grey levels or colour properties. Region-based methods are further categorized as region growing, region splitting, and merging. Now, we will discuss the region-growing method with an example in detail.

4.6 REGION-BASED METHODS

In region-based segmentation, we obtain some distinct regions or areas using homogeneity measures [16]. The partitioning may take place by checking the similarity in the neighbourhood and connecting with the adjacent pixels [17]. All the pixels are checked if the similarity exists with any of the segmented regions, and the method converges until no pixels are left to be partitioned, which means that all the pixels become part of some unique regions. The region-based method is of main two types: split and merge method, and region-growing method. The region-growing method is briefly explained here.

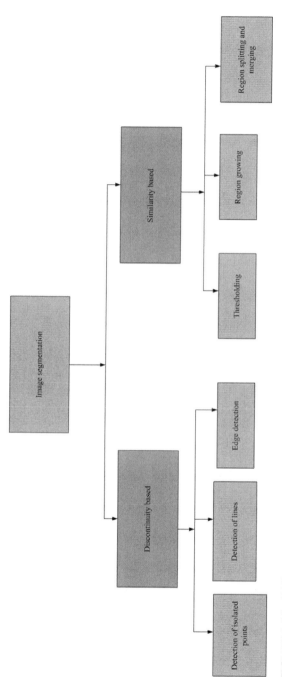

FIGURE 4.14　Different segmentation techniques used in Image processing.

4.6.1   REGION-GROWING SEGMENTATION

In the region-growing method, first a seed pixel is chosen and that pixel grows based on some similarity criterion which is evaluated with neighbourhood pixels [18]. The method can be easily understood with the help of the following major steps:

- Choose a seed point
- Select threshold value of the similarity metric (criterion)
- Evaluate the similarity criterion of the seed pixel with the pixels in the adjacent regions
- The pixels with similarity metrics lower than or equal to the threshold chosen, join with the seed pixel
- The seed grows until no other pixels meeting the criterion are left
- Start with other seed points
- Repeat the above steps until all the pixels are covered and the pixels become parts of some distinct regions

The ending of the segmentation is also termed convergence, under which no more segmentation is possible because all the pixels have been covered with the given seed pixels and criteria. The performance of segmentation, the segmentation result and convergence depend of the seed points, threshold values and the criteria selected in the method, and thus these factors affect the segmentation performance. The similarity metrics may be based on greyscale values, intensity, colour, gradient, mean of intensity and so on. We can see a sample result of segmentation using region growing for an original mammogram image, in Figure 4.15.

There are number of segmentation methods utilizing clustering approaches and fuzzy logic-based methods. Two sample results of fuzzy c-means (FCM) and k-means [19] [20] are shown in Figures 4.16 and 4.17 respectively [21].

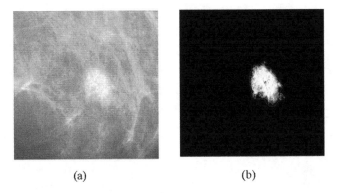

(a)   (b)

FIGURE 4.15   Region-growing segmentation (a) Original mammogram image (b) Segmented image.

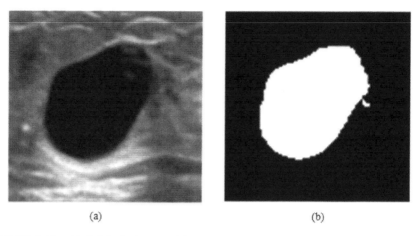

(a)   (b)

FIGURE 4.16   (a) Original ultrasound image of benign breast, (b) Result of segmentation using FCM.

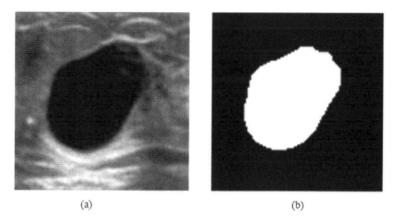

(a)   (b)

FIGURE 4.17   (a) Original ultrasound image of benign breast, (b) Result of segmentation using k-means.

FOLLOWING ARE ADVANTAGES AND DISADVANTAGES OF THE REGION-GROWING METHOD OF SEGMENTATION

ADVANTAGES

1. The region-growing technique can accurately separate the regions that have the same properties as defined.
2. This method can give good segmentation results for the original images with clear edges.
3. We can define the seed point and the criteria we want.

1. The main drawback of region growing is that manual interaction is needed for obtaining the seed point.
2. Oversegmentation or holes may result due to noise or intensity variation.

After completing this chapter, students/learners will be able to:

- Explain the significance of image enhancement and segmentation for medical image processing and applications
- Discuss a few practical examples of medical image enhancement and segmentation

LEARNING OUTCOMES

At the completion of this chapter, the students will be able to:

- Explain the medical image processing
- Discuss enhancement and segmentation necessary for medical image application

REFERENCES

1. Acharya, R., Wasserman, R., Stevens, J., & Hinojosa, C. (1995). Biomedical imaging modalities: a tutorial. *Computerized Medical Imaging and Graphics, 19*(1), 3–25.
2. Elangovan, A., & Jeyaseelan, T. (2016). Medical imaging modalities: A survey. In ICETETS, IEEE Staff (Ed.), *2016 International Conference on Emerging Trends in Engineering, Technology and Science* (pp. 1–4). IEEE.
3. Sagheer, S. V. M., & George, S. N. (2020). A review on medical image denoising algorithms. *Biomedical Signal Processing and Control, 61*, 102036.
4. Maini, R., & Aggarwal, H. (2010). A comprehensive review of image enhancement techniques. *Journal of Computing, 2*(3), 8–13.
5. Suckling, J. et al. (1994). The Mammographic Image Analysis Society digital mammogram database. *Exerpta Medica International Congress Series*, 375–378.
6. Patel, B. C., & Sinha, G. R. (2015). Gray level clustering and contrast enhancement (GLC–CE) of mammographic breast cancer images. *CSI Transactions on ICT, 2*(4), 279–286.
7. Gonzalez, R. C., & Woods, R. E. (2002). *Digital image processing.* Pearson Education.
8. Janani, P., Premaladha, J., & Ravichandran, K. S. (2015). Image enhancement techniques: A study. *Indian Journal of Science and Technology, 8*(22), 1–12.
9. Alisha, P. B., & Sheela, K. G. (2016). Image denoising techniques – an overview. *IOSR Journal of Electronics and Communication Engineering, 11*(1), 78–84.
10. Zhang, L., Chen, J., Zhu, Y., & Luo, J. (2009). Comparisons of several new denoising methods for medical images. In IEEE Engineering in Medicine and Biology Society (Ed.), *2009 3rd International Conference on Bioinformatics and Biomedical Engineering* (pp. 1–4). IEEE.
11. Patil, J., & Jadhav, S. (2013). A comparative study of image denoising techniques. *International Journal of Innovative Research in Science, Engineering and Technology, 2*(3), 787–794.

12. Rajni, R., & Anutam, A. (2014). Image denoising techniques – an overview. *International Journal of Computer Applications, 86*(16), 13–17.

13. Singh, B. K., Verma, K., & Thoke, A. S. (2015). Objective and optical evaluation of despeckle filters in breast ultrasound images. *IETE Technical Review, 32*(5), 384–398.

14. Fan, L., Zhang, F., Fan, H., & Zhang, C. (2019). Brief review of image denoising techniques. *Visual Computing for Industry, Biomedicine, and Art, 2*(1), 1–12.

15. Smistad, E., Falch, T. L., Bozorgi, M., Elster, A. C., & Lindseth, F. (2015). Medical image segmentation on GPUs – A comprehensive review. *Medical Image Analysis, 20*(1), 1–18.

16. Ghule, A. G., & Deshmukh, P. R. (2012). Image segmentation available techniques, open issues and region growing algorithm. *Journal of Signal and Image Processing, 3*(1), 71–75.

17. Norouzi, A., Rahim, M. S. M., Altameem, A., Saba, T., Rad, A. E., Rehman, A., & Uddin, M. (2014). Medical image segmentation methods, algorithms, and applications. *IETE Technical Review, 31*(3), 199–213.

18. Punitha, S., Ravi, S., & Devi, M. A. (2016). Breast cancer detection in digital mammograms using segmentation techniques. *International Journal of Circuit Theory and Applications, 9*(3), 167–182.

19. Singh, B. K., Jain, P., Banchhor, S. K., & Verma, K. (2019). Performance evaluation of breast lesion detection systems with expert delineations: a comparative investigation on mammographic images. *Multimedia Tools and Applications, 78*(16), 22421–22444.

20. Atrey, K., Singh, B. K., Roy, A., & Bodhey, N. K. (2020). Breast cancer detection and validation using dual modality imaging. In IEEED (Ed.), *2020 first international conference on power, control and computing technologies (ICPC2T)* (pp. 454–458). IEEE.

21. Al-Dhabyani W, Gomaa M, Khaled H, Fahmy A. (2020). Dataset of breast ultrasound images. *Data in Brief*, February, 104863. https://doi.org/10.1016/j.dib.2019.104863.

5 Bio-signals

LEARNING OBJECTIVES

- To understand an overview of bio-signals
- To get exposed to applications of different bio-signals

5.1 ORIGIN OF BIO-SIGNALS

The human body is a complex biological system that consists of various subsystems such as the respiration system, cardiovascular system, nervous system, digestive system and muscular system, which are used to perform a number of physiological activities to keep the body stable. Each subsystem has its own physiological process or physiological activity that can be measured in the form of a signal or chemical/hormonal reaction or physical form to study the state of the system. Any disease condition will disturb the physiological state of the system and that can be diagnosed with the help of bio-signals. Bio-signals are body-generated electrical potentials due to ionic movements within the cell [1]. There are different types of bio-signals in the human body which are associated to many physiological activities, explained in detail in following sections.

5.2 DIFFERENT TYPES OF BIO-SIGNALS

Different types of bio-signals used in the study of physiological studies are discussed in this section.

5.2.1 ELECTROCARDIOGRAM

An electrocardiogram (ECG) is the recording of electrical potentials generated by the contractile heart activity. ECG signals are recorded by placing surface electrodes on the chest and limb areas of the human body. This is one of the vital physiology parameters and thus the heartbeat can be measured by counting the peaks in the ECG waveforms. Many cardiovascular disorders can be analysed using ECG waveforms and their features because the morphology of the ECG alters with a pathological condition, which helps in detection and analysis of the disorder.

DOI: 10.1201/9781003097808-5

The human heart consists of four chambers – two atria and two ventricles. The atria collect the blood and the ventricles are responsible for the pumping of blood. These whole filling (diastole) and pumping (systole) activities of a heart correspond to one beat, or a cardiac cycle. The rhythmic activity of the heart is controlled by specialized pacemaker cells which form a sino-atrial node (SA node), and the firing rate of this node is managed by the central and autonomic nervous system impulses. The SA node is also known as a natural pacemaker of the heart that sends signals to the heart muscle, which further initiates the rhythmic contraction and expansion of heart muscles. The SA node fires or excites first, then the electrical potentials are passed to the atrial muscles, which causes the atrial muscles to depolarize slowly. This slow depolarization of the small atrial muscles results in the generation of slow P wave with less amplitude ranges 0.1–0.2 mV of about 60–80ms. After the P wave, the excited wave now faces ta transmission delay at the atrio-ventricular node of about 60–80 ms, and this delay helps in blood transferring from the atria to the ventricles; and this segment is known as the PQ segment. Now the excitatory wave spreads through the ventricles at a high rate through the bundle of His and Purkinje fibres, causing rapid ventricle depolarization. The depolarization of the ventricles generates a sharp biphasic or tri-phasic QRS wave amplitude around 1mV and a time duration of 80ms. After the QRS wave, there is a flat portion of action potential called as the ST segment with 100–120ms time duration. At the end, ventricular repolarization occurs, which generates a slow T wave of about 0.1–0.3 mV with 120–160ms of time duration [2]. This activity from P wave to T wave occurs during the contraction and expansion of the heart, which is known as the cardiac cycle, or heartbeat. Figure 5.1 shows the typical ECG signal waveform having a duration of three seconds.

The normal heart rate during the resting state is 70 beats per minute (bpm). A heart rate below 60 bpm at the rest state could possibly indicate the condition known as

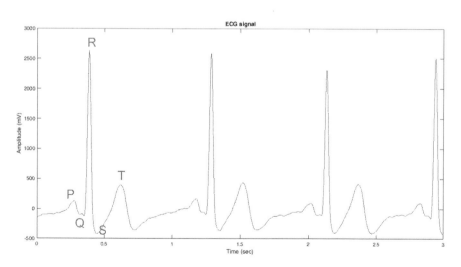

FIGURE 5.1   A typical ECG waveform.

bradycardia, and a heart rate above 150bpm at the rest state indicates an abnormal cardiac condition called tachycardia. Any abnormal heartbeat or abnormal SA firing or disturbance in the heartbeat is called cardiac arrhythmia.

ECG is considered one of the vital bio-signals which is used to analyse and detect the state of the heart and many cardiovascular diseases. Many cardiovascular diseases can specifically alter the ECG wave shape, which makes the ECG signal an important one in cardiovascular disease diagnosis.

The ECG signal is recorded using surface electrodes placed on the chest and limb areas. The ECG signal bandwidth is usually between 0.05Hz dan 100Hz. A clinical recording uses the standard 12-lead ECG systems where four limb electrodes and six chest electrodes are used. The four limb electrodes include the right arm, left arm, left leg and right leg, which are used to form Lead I, Lead II and Lead III connections to record the ECG. The right arm, left arm and left leg are connected to form a combined reference called the Wilson central terminal and used as a reference for chest lead connections. Figure 5.2 shows the Einthoven's triangle and the connection for six limb electrodes. The aVR, aVL and aVF in Figure 5.2 denote the augmented limb connection for the right arm, left arm and left leg respectively where the active limb electrodes are referenced to Wilson's central terminal.

Other than limb electrodes, there are six chest electrodes V1 to V6 placed at six standard positions on chest areas referenced to Wilson's central terminal. The 12-lead ECG (which includes six limb and six chest electrodes) recording is standardized practice in clinics, and the interpretations are drawn purely based on empirical and

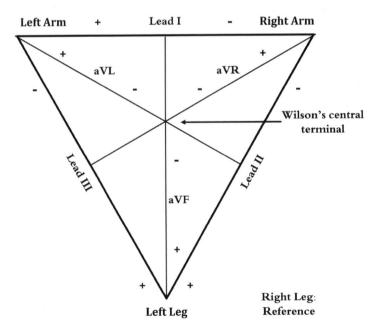

FIGURE 5.2 ECG leads and Einthoven triangle.

experimental knowledge. The relationships between ECG leads are given in Equations (5.1) and (5.2):

$$\text{Lead II} = \text{Lead I} + \text{Lead III} \tag{5.1}$$

$$\text{aVL} = (\text{I} - \text{III}) / 2 \tag{5.2}$$

5.2.2 ELECTROENCEPHALOGRAM (EEG)

The EEG is the recording of the electrical activity of the brain. The different brain regions generate electrical signals corresponding to its specific functions and those signals may be recorded using surface electrodes at the scalp. The scalp EEG is the summation of a post-synaptic response generated by the firing of millions of neurons synchronously under the electrode. A clinical EEG uses recordings from several channels at different brain areas on the scalp and performs a comparative analysis of brain activation from different brain regions. For a clinical EEG recording, a standard 10–20 electrode placement method (see Figure 5.3) has been recommended by the International Federation of Societies for Electroencephalography and Clinical Neurophysiology.

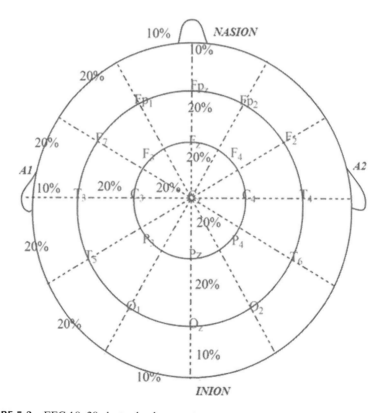

FIGURE 5.3   EEG 10–20 electrode placement.

As the name indicates, the electrodes are placed at a distance of 10, 20, 20, 20, 20 and 10% from the total distance between nasion and inion. The brain areas are divided into the prefrontal, frontal, central, parietal, temporal and occipital lobes. The electrode placement follows symmetric positioning, and the electrodes in the left hemisphere of brain are denoted by odd number and the electrodes in the right hemisphere by even numbers. In general, EEG signal bandwidth ranges from 0.1 to 100 Hz and is divided into various sub-bands or brain rhythms (see Figure 5.4) such as:

- Delta (0.1–4 Hz),
- Theta (4–8 Hz),
- Alpha (8–14 Hz) and
- Beta (14–30 Hz).

Each EEG rhythm has its own clinical importance associated to brain functions. The alpha wave is generally seen during wakeful rest and in resting adults in the occipital areas. The alpha wave is dominant during auditory processing and arithmetic processing with a closed-eyes condition and starts to decrease when the eyes open. The alpha waves are occupied by slower waves at various sleep stages. The theta wave is seen primarily at the beginning of sleep and replaced by the delta wave at deep sleep stages. The synchronization or desynchronization of any wave during any specific task may indicate a possible abnormal condition of the brain [2]. For example, the increase of delta during any cognitive task or at wakeful rest in adults could indicate an abnormal condition. EEG signals have been largely used in clinical research and in various disease diagnoses including epilepsy [3], schizophrenia [4], Parkinson [5], dyslexia [6], dementia [7] and other similar brain disorders and disabilities. EEG signals are also used in the study of various psychological and cognitive aspects of the human brain.

5.2.3 Electroocculogram (EOG)

EOG is a method of recording the standing corneo-retinal electrical potential that exists between the front and back of the eye [8]. The EOG signal measures the potential difference between the positive cornea potential and the negative cornea potential, simply called corneo-retinal potential. EOG signals have low frequency with amplitude value ranging from 0.3 to 1mV and are widely used with EEG recording to remove the eye-blink and the eye movement artefacts in EEG recording. In recent times, EOG signals have been used in human computer interface (HCI) where eye movements control cursor movements. Along with the electroretinogram (ERG), EOG signals are used to confirm the presence of the diseases (egg-yellow fundus) [8]. EOG signals are recorded by placing electrodes beside the eye, and the ground electrode is placed on the forehead or earlobe. Figure 5.5 shows the recorded EOG signals for 20 seconds.

5.2.4 Electromyogram (EMG)

EMG signals represent electrical signals that are produced due to the contraction of muscles when the muscle cells are externally or neurologically affected. The

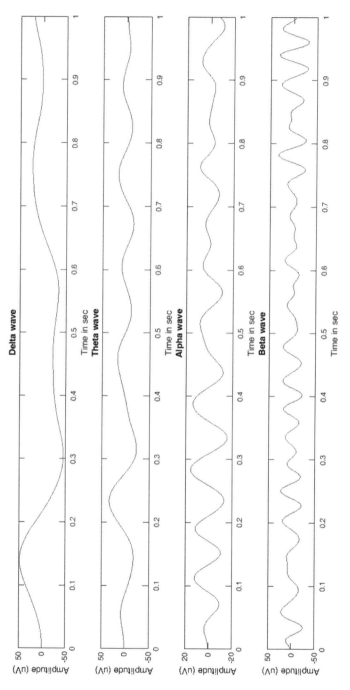

FIGURE 5.4 EEG bands.

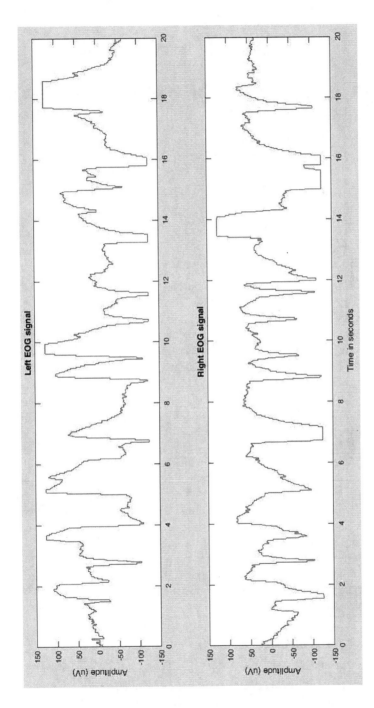

FIGURE 5.5 EOG signal [9].

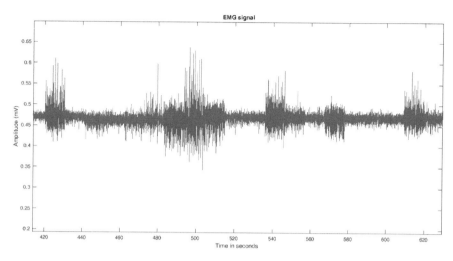

FIGURE 5.6   EMG signal.

electrical potential is developed within muscle cells when the depolarization and repolarization of muscles occurs and passes all over the muscle fibres. The skeletal muscles are collections of many motor units (MUs). An MU is the smallest unit in the muscles and the contraction of an MU generates an electrical signal when excited by a neural signal. The generated electrical signal is the single motor unit action potential (SMUAP), which can be recorded using needle electrodes over the area of interest. The amplitude of the normal SMUAP varies from 100 to 400 microvolts with 6–30 Hz frequency range [2]. The recorded SMUAP signal shape depends on the type of needle used and the recording site with respect to an active MU. Any diseased condition alters the shape of the SMUAP. Neuropathy causes reduced activation and conduction in muscle fibres, which leads to poly-phasic SMUAP (unusual higher amplitude level than normal). Myopathy causes muscle fibre loss within MUs along with intact neurons. Muscular activation and contraction are generally controlled by spatial and temporal recruitment of MUs. In spatial recruitment, new MUs are activated with increasing effort and in temporal recruitment, and the firing rate for each MU is increased with increasing effort. An asynchronous contraction of an MU occurs due to asynchronous firing of the MU at different frequency and times. The summation SMUAP from all active MUs gives rise to an EMG signal. Figure 5.6 shows the EMG signals recorded using surface electrodes. An EMG signal represents the level of muscle activation at the recording site and used in the diagnosis of many neuromuscular diseases.

5.3   NOISE AND ARTEFACTS

Most biomedical signals are generally weak in nature and mixed with many unwanted sources. Any recorded signals other than those of our interest are called artefacts or noises. The unwanted signals which are referred to as noise or artefacts are contributed by a number of sources, including powerline. The noises in the bio-signal may be due to various factors [10], such as

- Physiological artefacts
- Instrumentation artefacts
- Environmental artefacts
- Motion artefacts

Physiological artefacts – The human body possesses various physiological systems which generate various electrical signals at any given time related to its activity. So any signal that is added to the recording other than our signal of interest is termed physiological interference. These artefacts are dynamic and non-stationary in nature as they do not show any specific pattern or fixed frequency content. A few examples are

- Eyeblinks, EMG and ECG artefacts in EEG recording,
- Maternal ECG artefacts in fetal ECG and
- Lung sound and respiration sound mixed with heart sound.

Instrumentation artefacts – Most bio-signals are weak in nature and need amplification to detect or to record meaningful information. The amplification gain factor may vary from a hundreds to thousands level, and in each level the electronic noise in the amplifier will also get amplified along with the bio-signal. The instrumentation noise can be nullified by using modern electronic devices with low-noise power, high common mode rejection and high-input impedance for signal acquisition.

Environmental artefacts – The major source for environmental noise is the electromagnetic (EM) waves around us. The EM waves emitted from a device such as a radio, television towers, monitors and other devices in the lab environment may be picked up by recording devices and cables. Also, 50/60 Hz powerline interference may get added to the recording and corrupt the bio-signal. Powerline interference is the most common interference from the recording environment and it is periodic in nature and has a fixed frequency spectrum. The usage of proper EM-shielded cables and proper grounding of the device may reduce powerline interference and EM interference to the recording.

Motion or movement artefacts – Motion or movement artefacts are due to the subject movement or lead movement at the time of recording. During recording, the bio-signal may get affected when the subject moves or the electrode position changes, and it produces a large spike or peak with amplitude relatively larger than the actual bio-signal.

5.4 FILTERING OF BIO-SIGNALS

The quality of bio-signals is badly affected by noise, which can be reduced by using suitable filters. Filtering is the process of removing a signal of no interest (artefacts/noises) from the desired or recorded signal. Filtering of bio-signals is one of the vital procedure in bio-signal processing as most bio-signals recorded in a clinical envir-onment are contaminated with noise. Such interference or noise alters the signal of interest and makes it difficult to extract useful or actual information about the bio-signal. So, the filtering of noises in bio-signals is required to enhance the quality of the signal and therefore it helps in an accurate diagnosis. On the basis of how filters modify the signal spectrum, it can be broadly classified into three classes, namely high-pass, low-pass and band-pass filters [11]. Low-pass filters keep the selected low-frequency components and remove the high-frequency components in the desired signal, whereas the high-pass filter allows the high-frequency components and suppresses the low-frequency components in the signal. The band-pass filter and band-stop filter in other terms keeps only the selected band (in band-pass) or removes the selected band (in band-stop) of frequencies and suppresses the frequencies which fall less or beyond the selected range of frequencies. Band-pass/band-stop filters are simply obtained by combining low-pass and high-pass filters. The above-discussed filters work well only when the signal spectrum and noise spectrum are different. But in the real-time recording of bio-signals, the noise spectrum gets overlapped with the bio-signal spectrum. In such cases, the traditional filters may not be successful in removing the noise in the signal. In real time, most bio-signals are considered to be the sum of the actual signal and noise component, as given in Equation (5.3):

$$x_n(t) = x(t) + n(t). \qquad (5.3)$$

The signal $x_n(t)$ represents the recorded signal at n^{th} trial which contains the desired signal $x(t)$ and the noise component $n(t)$. Most noises which contaminate the bio-signal are random in nature. In such a case, signal averaging will help in reducing the noises and provides a close approximation of the true bio-signal. Signal averaging may be done in both the time and frequency domain, which depends on the nature of the signal. Signal averaging in the frequency domain is preferable for signals which are random in nature. In recent times, many advanced signal filtering techniques such as adaptive filtering [12], wavelet de-noising [13], principal component analysis [14], and independent component analysis [14] techniques are used in bio-signal processing.

5.5   APPLICATIONS OF BIO-SIGNALS

Various types of bio-signals are used for numerous applications, especially in bio-medical and cognitive science applications [15–21]. The cognitive abilities of the human brain, motor imagery task classification, workload assessment and many others, in addition to research and the study of brain disorders are application areas where bio-signals are utilized. There are datasets available as open source that can be used by researchers for biomedical applications.

LEARNING OUTCOME

After reading this chapter, students and readers will be able to:

• Explain various types of bio-signals with their usage

REFERENCES

1. Kaniusas, E. (2012). Fundamentals of biosignals. In *Biomedical signals and sensors I* (pp. 1–26). Springer.
2. Rangayyan, R. M. (2015). *Biomedical signal analysis*. John Wiley.
3. Mandal, S., Thakur, M., Thakur, K., & Singh, B. K. (2020). Comparative investigation of different classification techniques for epilepsy detection using EEG signals. In A. A., Rizvanov, B. K. Singh, & P. Ganasala (Eds.), *Advances in Biomedical Engineering and Technology. Lecture Notes in Bioengineering* (pp. 413–424). Springer. https://doi.org/10.1007/978-981-15-6329-4_34
4. Tikka, S. K. et al. (2020). Artificial intelligence-based classification of schizophrenia: A high density electroencephalographic and support vector machine study. *Indian Journal of Psychiatry, 62*(3), 273–282.
5. Klassen, B. T. et al. (2011). Quantitative EEG as a predictive biomarker for Parkinson disease dementia. *Neurology, 77*(2), 118–124.
6. Seshadri, N. P. G., Geethanjali, B., & Singh, B. K. (2020). Resting state EEG signal analysis in Indian dyslexic children. In *2020 First International Conference on Power, Control and Computing Technologies (ICPC2T)* (pp. 300–304). IEEE.
7. Adler, G., Brassen, S., & Jajcevic, A. (2003). EEG coherence in Alzheimer's dementia. *Journal of Neural Transmission, 110*(9), 1051–1058.
8. Creel, D. J. (2019). The electrooculogram. *Handbook of Clinical Neurology, 160*, 495–499. https://doi.org/10.1016/B978-0-444-64032-1.00033-3
9. Goldberger, A., Amaral, L., Glass, J., Hausdorff, J., Ivanov, P. C., Mark, R., … & Stanley, H. E. (2003). PhysioBank, PhysioToolkit, and PhysioNet: Components of a new research resource for complex physiologic signals. *Circulation* Online, *101*(23), e215–e220.
10. Srivastava, S., & Jain, S. (2020). Optimum digital filter design for removal of different noises from biomedical signals. In N. Marriwala, C. C. Tripathi, D. Kumar, & S. Jain (Eds.), *Mobile Radio Communications and 5G Networks. Lecture Notes in Networks and Systems* (Vol. 140, pp. 389–399). Springer.
11. Escabí, M. A. (2005). Biosignal processing. In John D. Enderle, Susan M. Blanchard, & Joseph D. Bronzino (Eds.), *Introduction to biomedical engineering* (2nd ed.) (pp. 549–625). Academic Press. https://doi.org/10.1016/B978-0-12-238662-6.50012-4
12. Smital, L., Vitek, M., Kozumplík, J., & Provaznik, I. (2012). Adaptive wavelet wiener filtering of ECG signals. *IEEE Transactions on Biomedical Engineering, 60*(2), 437–445.
13. Poornachandra, S. (2008). Wavelet-based denoising using subband dependent threshold for ECG signals. *Digital Signal Processing, 18*(1), 49–55.
14. Romero, I. (2011). PCA and ICA applied to noise reduction in multi-lead ECG. *2011 Computing in Cardiology*, 613–616. https://ieeexplore.ieee.org/document/6164640
15. Bajaj, V., & Sinha, G. R. (2021). *Computer-aided design and diagnosis methods for biomedical applications*. CRC Press.
16. Bajaj, V., & Sinha, G. R. (2020). *Modelling and analysis of active bio-potential signals in healthcare* (Vol. 1). IOP Publishing.
17. Bajaj, V., & Sinha, G. R. (2020). *Modelling and analysis of active bio-potential signals in healthcare* (Vol. 2). IOP Publishing.
18. Taran, S., Bajaj, V., Sinha, G. R., & Polat, K. (2021). Detection of sleep apnea events using electroencephalogram signals. *Applied Acoustics, 181*, 108137, https://doi.org/10.1016/j.apacoust.2021.108137.

19. Mohdiwale, S., Sahu, M., Sinha, G. R., & Bhateja, V. (2021). Statistical wavelets with harmony search-based optimal feature selection of EEG signals for motor imagery classification. *IEEE Sensors Journal, 21*(13), 14263–14271. https://doi.org/10.1109/JSEN.2020.3026172.

20. Khare, S. K., Bajaj, V., & Sinha, G. R. (2020). Adaptive tunable Q wavelet transform-based emotion identification. *IEEE Transactions on Instrumentation and Measurement, 69*(12), 9609–9617. https://doi.org/ 10.1109/TIM.2020.3006611.

21. Samrudhi Mohdiwale, M. S., Sinha, G. R., & Bajaj, V. (2020). Automated cognitive workload assessment using logical teaching learning based optimization and PROMETHEE multi-criteria decision making approach. *IEEE Sensor Journal, 20*(22), 13629–13637. https://ieeexplore.ieee.org/document/9131752.

6 Feature Extraction

LEARNING OBJECTIVES

This chapter aims to cover:

- Image feature extraction related to texture and shape
- Feature normalization

After pre-processing and noise removal from medical images, the next step is to extract suitable features to represent and distinguish normal and abnormal regions or tissues. Feature is a function of one or more measurements which quantifies some significant characteristics of an object. In general, feature extraction is an essential step in computer-aided diagnosis (CAD) of medical images.

6.1 FEATURE EXTRACTION

Once the pre-processing and image enhancement are applied to the images, the next step is to extract suitable features which indicate the information of images used for further stages. For example, in breast cancer detection, benign and malignant tissues need to be clearly identified that can be easily distinguished by shape- and texture-based features of the selected regions. Simple to complex patterns present in medical images need to be interpreted for automated analysis of images, and this requires features that can be extracted using suitable feature extraction methods. Based on image modality, the types of features may be different, whether shape-based features, texture-based features or some statistical features derived from images or other features. The features are utilized for classification or prediction purposes, and thus features are subjected to classifiers, but before classification feature normalization is applied, and then normalized features are given as input to the classifier. Normalization can also be implemented by using a suitable computational algorithm or method, and appropriate normalization is needed so that proper structure and information are obtained for classification and post-processing of the images.

In this chapter, texture and shape-based features extracted from medical images are discussed with their extraction methods. The effect of these features used in various classifiers, is also assessed.

DOI: 10.1201/9781003097808-6

6.2 ECHOGRAPHIC CHARACTERISTICS OF BREAST TUMOURS IN ULTRASOUND IMAGING

To understand the importance of texture and shape features in medical image processing, consider the tissues in ultrasound images of the breast. We can see texture- and shape-based features that help in differentiating the tissues as malignant and benign. The following criteria are important in the procedure of obtaining the characteristics:

a. The internal echo patterns of tumour in the breast are either heterogeneous or homogeneous, both for malignant and benign masses [1, 2], as shown in Figure 6.1. The texture feature or metrics are used for modelling the echo patterns.
b. Generally, the tumour is seen as oval, round or in some other irregular shape. Regular shapes such as oval and round are benign masses, and malignant masses exhibit irregular shapes [2, 3]. The shapes and their measurements can be made using parameters such as area, perimeter, compactness and so on.
c. Lesions present in the breast are of isoechoic, hyperechoic, hypoechoic or anechoic types. A benign cyst shows an anechoic lesion, and a hypoechoic lesion seems to be fat in its surrounding, which indicates a malignant mass. The hyperechogenic lesion is generally benign in nature [1, 4].

6.3 TEXTURE FEATURE EXTRACTION

A number of approaches to extracting texture and shape information have been developed over the years. The texture of an image can be defined as spatial distribution of grey levels over the pixels in an image [5]. It is one of the important characteristics used in identifying objects or a region of interest (ROI) in an image. It is a property of areas; that is, the texture of a point is undefined. So, texture is a contextual property and its definition must involve grey values in a spatial neighbourhood. The size of the neighbourhood depends upon the texture type or the size of the primitives defining the texture [6]. Texture has multiple dimensions. Hence, there is no single method of texture representation, which can be used to characterize a variety of textures. Various texture features that can be extracted are the following:

6.3.1 First-Order Statistical Features

A grey value at some random location can be observed and first-order statistics can be measured. This can be done directly from grey-scale values of the original images without taking neighbourhood pixels into consideration [7]. First-order statistics are generally derived from a first-order histogram of the image. A histogram of intensity levels is a simple summary of the statistical information of the image. The first-order histogram $P(I)$ of an image is defined as:

$$P(I) = \frac{N(I)}{N}, \tag{6.1}$$

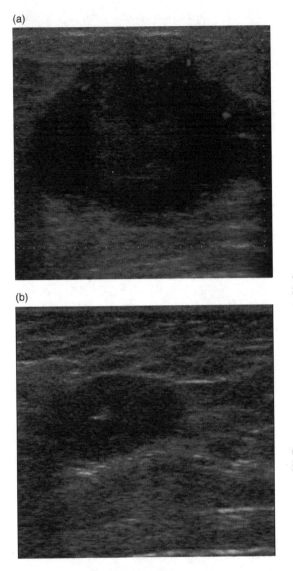

FIGURE 6.1 Breast ultrasound image containing (a) malignant tumour and (b) benign tumour.

where $N(I)$ is the number of pixels with grey-level I, and N is the total number of pixels in the region. If L is the total number of possible grey levels in the image, various features that can be derived from this approach are [8]:

a. *Mean (m)*: It is a measure of average intensity of the image. It is given by:

$$m = \sum_{I=0}^{L-1} IP(I), \qquad (6.2)$$

where I is the random variable representing the grey levels in ROI.

b. *Variance* (μ_2): It is a measure of width of the histogram; that is, it measures how much the grey levels differ from the mean. It is calculated using:

$$\mu_2 = \sigma^2 = \sum_{I=0}^{L-1}(I-m)^2 P(I). \tag{6.3}$$

c. *Standard deviation* (σ): It is the measure of average contrast of an image. It is calculated using:

$$\sigma = \sqrt{\mu_2}. \tag{6.4}$$

d. *Skewness* (μ_3): It is a measure of the degree of histogram asymmetry around the mean. For a symmetric histogram, it tends to be zero; otherwise, its value is positive or negative depending upon whether the histogram is skewed to the right or left respectively. This is illustrated in Figure 6.2. It is computed using:

$$\mu_3 = \sum_{I=0}^{L-1}(I-m)^3 P(I). \tag{6.5}$$

e. *Kurtosis* (μ_4): Kurtosis is a measure of sharpness of the image. Its value is low for a sharp histogram (leptokurtic) and high for a spread histogram (platykurtic) [9]. This is illustrated in Figure 6.3.

$$\mu_4 = \sum_{I=0}^{L-1}(I-m)^4 P(I). \tag{6.6}$$

f. *Measure of smoothness (R)*: A measure of smoothness R is determined using:

$$R = 1 - \frac{1}{1+\sigma^2}. \tag{6.7}$$

The value of R is zero for a region of constant intensity and approaches one for a region with large excursions in the values of its intensity levels.

g. *Measure of uniformity (U)*: It is given by:

$$U = \sum_{I=0}^{L-1} P^2(I). \tag{6.8}$$

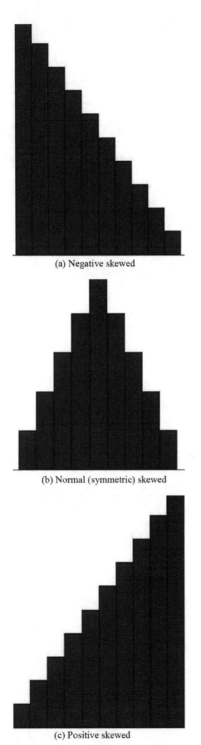

(a) Negative skewed

(b) Normal (symmetric) skewed

(c) Positive skewed

FIGURE 6.2 Illustration of skewness. (a) Negative skewed, (b) Normal (symmetric) and (c) Positive skewed.

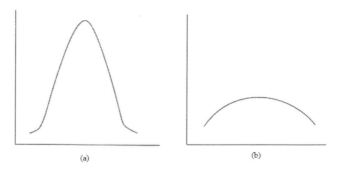

(a)   (b)

FIGURE 6.3   Illustration of kurtosis. (a) Leptokurtic and (b) Platykurtic.

The uniformity measure U attains a maximum value when all the grey levels are equal (maximally uniform).

h. *Entropy (E)*: Entropy measures the histogram uniformity. It is calculated using:

$$E = \sum_{I=0}^{L-1} P(I) \log_2 P(I). \tag{6.9}$$

A higher value of uniformity results in higher entropy.

Though simple to calculate, texture analysis based solely on a grey-level histogram suffers from the limitation that it provides no information about the relative position of various grey levels within the image [9, 10].

6.3.2   GREY-LEVEL CO-OCCURRENCE MATRICES

The relative postions of the pixels in images are ignored by first-order statistics and this can be overcome by using grey-level co-occurrence (GLC) texture features, as suggested by [5, 10–12]. The GLC matrix, also called GLCM, considers the second-order joint probability density function $f(i, j; d, \theta)$. The GLCM is also referred to as spatial GLCM (SGLCM), in which relative frequency is indicated by each entry with respect to two neighbouring cells having grey-scale values i and j respectively. The distance d and orientation θ are used to separate the two resolution cells. The orientation is further quantized as horizontal, diagonal, vertical and antidiagonal directions $(0^0, 45^0, 90^0, and 135^0)$, as shown in Figure 6.4. Given an image $I(m, n)$, for fixed d, each entry N (say) in $f(i, j; d, \theta)$ for various values of θ is defined as:

$$0^0: N\,(I(m,\,n) = I_1,\, I(m \pm d,\, n) = I_2), \tag{6.10}$$

$$45^0: N\,(I(m,\,n) = I_1,\, I(m \pm d,\, n \mp d) = I_2), \tag{6.11}$$

$$90^0: N\,(I(m,\,n) = I_1,\, I(m,\, n \mp d) = I_2), \tag{6.12}$$

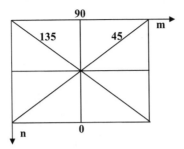

FIGURE 6.4 The four orientations used to construct co-occurrence matrices.

$$135^\circ: N\,(I(m,\,n) = I_1,\, I(m \pm d,\, n \pm d) = I_2), \tag{6.13}$$

where N is the number of pairs of pixels at distance d with values $(I_1,\, I_2)$.
For example, consider a 3×3 image matrix $I(m,\, n)$:

$$I = \begin{bmatrix} 1 & 0 & 2 \\ 1 & 1 & 2 \\ 0 & 2 & 1 \end{bmatrix}. \tag{6.14}$$

The grey levels of image I lie from zero to maximum up to two; that is, the image I is quantized into three discrete grey levels, say denoted by L ($L = 3$). The co-occurrence matrix for a pair $(d,\, \theta)$ will be an $L \times L$ matrix of the following structure:

$$f = \begin{bmatrix} N(0,0) & N(0,1) & N(0,2) \\ N(1,0) & N(1,1) & N(1,2) \\ N(2,0) & N(2,1) & N(2,2) \end{bmatrix}, \tag{6.15}$$

where $N(I_1,\, I_2)$ is the number of pixel pairs, at relative position $(d,\, \theta)$, which have grey-level values $I_1,\, I_2,$ respectively. For the image I represented by equation 4.14, the following co-occurrence matrices are obtained:

$$f(1, 0^0) = \begin{bmatrix} 0 & 1 & 2 \\ 1 & 2 & 2 \\ 2 & 2 & 0 \end{bmatrix}, \tag{6.16}$$

$$f(1, 90^0) = \begin{bmatrix} 0 & 2 & 0 \\ 2 & 2 & 2 \\ 2 & 2 & 2 \end{bmatrix}, \tag{6.17}$$

$$f(1,45^0) = \begin{bmatrix} 0 & 2 & 0 \\ 2 & 0 & 1 \\ 0 & 1 & 2 \end{bmatrix}, \tag{6.18}$$

$$f(1,135^0) = \begin{bmatrix} 0 & 0 & 1 \\ 0 & 4 & 1 \\ 1 & 1 & 0 \end{bmatrix}. \tag{6.19}$$

It is a noteworthy point that certain pairs of grey-level co-occurrence matrices are symmetric to each other [5]. In particular, the relationship $f(i, j; d, \theta) = f(j, i; d, \theta)$ exists between two grey-level co-occurrence matrices. If the estimated probability distribution is denoted by $f(d, \theta)$, and $f'(d, \theta)$ denotes its transpose, the following relations hold true:

$$f(d, 0^0) = f'(d, 180^0),$$

$$f(d, 45^0) = f'(d, 225^0),$$

$$f(d, 90^0) = f'(d, 270^0),$$

$$f(d, 135^0) = f'(d, 315^0). \tag{6.20}$$

Thus, the knowledge of $f(d, 180^0)$, $f(d, 225^0)$, $f(d, 270^0)$, and $f(d, 315^0)$ does not contribute additionally to the texture pattern. After obtaining the co-occurrence matrix, the following texture features are extracted:

a. *Angular second moment (ASM):*

$$ASM = \sum_{i=1}^{L} \sum_{j=1}^{L} \left(f(i, j)^2 \right) \tag{6.21}$$

b. *Contrast (CON):*

$$CON = \sum_{n=0}^{L-1} n^2 \left\{ \sum_{i=1}^{L} \sum_{j=1}^{L} f(i, j) \right\}, \text{where } n = |i - j| \tag{6.22}$$

c. *Correlation (COR):*

$$COR = \frac{\sum_{i=1}^{L} \sum_{j=1}^{L} (ij) f(i, j) - \mu_x \mu_y}{\sigma_x \sigma_y}, \tag{6.23}$$

where μ_x, μ_y, σ_x and σ_y are the means and standard deviations of f_x and f_y respectively.

d. *Sum of squares variance (SOSV):*

$$SOSV = \sum_{i=1}^{L}\sum_{j=1}^{L}(i-\mu)^2 f(i,j) \tag{6.24}$$

e. *Inverse difference moment (IDM):*

$$IDM = \sum_{i=1}^{L}\sum_{j=1}^{L}\frac{1}{1+(i-j)^2}f(i,j) \tag{6.25}$$

f. *Sum average (SA):*

$$SA = \sum_{i=2}^{2L} if_{x+y}(i), \tag{6.26}$$

where

$$f_{x+y}(k) = \sum_{i=1}^{L}\sum_{j=1}^{L}f(i,j), i+j = k \text{ and } k = 2, 3,\ldots\ldots,2L. \tag{6.27}$$

g. *Sum variance (SV):*

$$SV = \sum_{i=2}^{2L}(i-SE)^2 f_{x+y}(i) \tag{6.28}$$

h. *Sum entropy (SE):*

$$SE = -\sum_{i=2}^{2L}f_{x+y}(i)\log\left\{f_{x+y}(i)\right\} \tag{6.29}$$

i. *Entropy (E):*

$$E = -\sum_{i=1}^{L}\sum_{j=1}^{L}f(i,j)\log(f(i,j)) \tag{6.30}$$

j. *Difference variance (DV)*:

$$DV = Variance\ of\ f_{x-y},\tag{6.31}$$

where

$$f_{x-y}(k) = \sum_{i=1}^{L}\sum_{j=1}^{L} f(i,j), |i-j| = k\ and\ k = 0,1,\ldots\ldots,2L\tag{6.32}$$

k. *Difference entropy (DE)*: It is calculated using:

$$DE = -\sum_{i=0}^{L-1} f_{x-y}(i)\log\left\{f_{x-y}(i)\right\}\tag{6.33}$$

l. *Information measures of correlation 1 (IM1)*:

$$IM1 = \frac{H_{XY} - H_{XY1}}{\max\left\{H_x H_y\right\}}\tag{6.34}$$

m. *Information measures of correlation 2 (IM2)*:

$$IM2 = \sqrt{\left(1 - \exp\left[-2(H_{XY2} - H_{XY})\right]\right)},\tag{6.35}$$

where H_{XY} = E (Entropy), H_x and H_y are entropies of f_x and f_y respectively, and H_{XY1} and H_{XY2} are calculated using:

$$H_{XY1} = -\sum_{i=0}^{L-1}\sum_{j=0}^{L-1} f(i,j)\log(f_x(i),f_y(j))\ and\tag{6.36}$$

$$H_{XY2} = -\sum_{i=0}^{L-1}\sum_{j=0}^{L-1} f_x(i),f_y(j)\log(f_x(i),f_y(j)).\tag{6.37}$$

The marginal probability matrices $f_x(i)$ and $f_y(j)$ are obtained by summing the rows and columns of $f(i,j)$ respectively using the following equations:

$$f_x(i) = \sum_{j=1}^{L} f(i,j)\tag{6.38}$$

$$f_y(j) = \sum_{i=1}^{L} f(i, j).$$ (6.39)

The above features, either all or some of them, are used in various applications depending upon the imaging modalities employed and their interpretation requirement. The important point to be taken care of is the high discriminatory nature of features. For example, ASM will be larger for a homogeneous image while smaller for a non-homogenous one. The feature CON measures the amount of local variations in the image. Hence, its value will be higher for a good contrast image or an image with a higher amount of local variations. All these features are a function of orientation and distance. Therefore, the features differ upon rotating the image, which is not useful to have a robust interpretation of the image, and their usefulness does not remain good so as to employ the features for robust image interpretation.. So, the distance is considered as average involving the values in all four directions so as make texture features rotation invariant.

6.3.3 GREY-LEVEL DIFFERENCE STATISTICS

The third category of useful texture features are those obtained from the statistics of local property values. These statistics are called grey-level difference statistics (GLDS), proposed in [11]. In this technique, local properties such as mean, contrast and so on, based on absolute differences between pairs of grey levels or average grey levels, are computed. Let us consider image $F(x, y)$ for which GLDS are to be calculated. For any given displacement δ, let $F_\delta(x, y) = |F(x, y) - F(x + \delta x, y + \delta y)|$ and p_δ be the probability density of $F_\delta(x, y)$. If there are L distinct grey levels, then, p_δ is a one-dimensional vector whose i^{th} component is the probability that $F_\delta(x, y)$ will have the value i [11, 12]. Assuming the image texture as coarse, having a lower value of δ, especially in comparison with the size of the texture element, grey levels will be smaller in different pairs of points for the separation value of δ. Hence, there will be low values for $F_\delta(x, y)$ and the values will be concentrated to I = 0 for the values in $p_\delta(i)$. On the other hand, the spread will be more for finer texture values [11, 12]. In this work, p_δ is calculated for four different orientations (0^0, 45^0, 90^0, and 135^0) and $\delta = 1$. The resulting values for the four directions are averaged out so as to make texture features rotation invariant. After obtaining p_δ, the following four texture measures are calculated:

a. *Contrast (CON)*:

$$CON = \sum i^2 p_\delta(i)$$ (6.40)

b. *Angular second moment (ASM)*:

$$ASM = \sum p_\delta(i)^2$$ (6.41)

c. *Entropy (E)*:

$$E = -\sum p_\delta(i) \log p_\delta(i) \tag{6.42}$$

d. *Mean*:

$$Mean = \left(\frac{1}{L}\right) \sum i p_\delta(i). \tag{6.43}$$

The value of ASM is smallest when the values in $p_\delta(i)$ are all as equal as possible, and large when some values in $p_\delta(i)$ are high and others are low. E is largest for equal values in $p_\delta(i)$ and small when the values in $p_\delta(i)$ are very different. Mean is small when values in $p_\delta(i)$ are concentrated near the origin, while large when they are far from the origin.

6.3.4   Neighbourhood Grey-Tone Difference Matrix

The visual contents of images are expressed as texture features, which are very useful in medical image analysis and diagnosis processes [13]. For selecting a ROI, we check the intensity variation in the neighbourhood, and pixel grey-scale variations are observed and accordingly the texture is estimated as the measure of grey-level tones of the surrounding neighbours of various pixels. For each of the elected ROIs, we chose a 1D matrix where the ith entry indicates the sum of the difference between the adjacent grey levels evaluated for all pixels having the grey-level i and the mean level of the surrounding pixels. This matrix is known as the neighbourhood grey-tone difference matrix (NGTDM). The size of the neighbourhood depends on the selected distance, that is, a distance equal to one result in a 3 × 3 neighbourhood [14]. Let $I[m,n]$ be the image matrix having a grey tone i at some value of $[m, n]$. Then the average grey tone over the neighbourhood is centred at i, but excluding i is given by:

$$\overline{A_i} = \overline{A(m,n)} = \frac{1}{w-1}\left[\sum_{x=-d}^{d}\sum_{y=-d}^{d} I(m+x, n+y)\right], (x,y) \neq (0,0), \tag{6.44}$$

where d specifies the neighbourhood size and $w = (2d + 1)^2$. The ith entry in the NGTDM is given by:

$$s(i) = \sum \left|i - \overline{A_i}\right|, \text{for } i \in N_i \text{ if } N_i \neq 0,$$
$$= 0, \textit{otherwise}, \tag{6.45}$$

where N_i is the set of all pixels having a grey tone i (except in the peripheral regions of width d). To illustrate the calculation of the NGTDM, consider a 5 × 5 image matrix $I(m, n)$:

$$I = \begin{bmatrix} 1 & 1 & 4 & 2 & 1 \\ 1 & 3^* & 5^* & 2^* & 3 \\ 2 & 2^* & 3^* & 5^* & 2 \\ 3 & 1^* & 2^* & 3^* & 1 \\ 1 & 2 & 4 & 1 & 5 \end{bmatrix}. \tag{6.46}$$

If the value of $d = 1$, then a 3×3 neighbourhood will be considered for obtaining the NGTDM. Further, this neighbourhood can only be centred on pixels marked "*". The remaining pixels are assumed to be on the periphery of the image. The pixels marked "*" are assigned grey tone 5. So, for such an image:

$$s(5) = \left| 5 - \frac{22}{8} \right| + \left| 5 - \frac{21}{8} \right| = 2.250 + 2.375 = 4.625 \, (6.46a) \text{ Similarly}$$

$$s(1) = 1.375, s(2) = 1.125 + 0.5 + 0.625 = 2.25, s(3)$$
$$= 0.625 + 0.125 + 0.125 = 0.875, s(4) = 0.$$

Thus, the NGTDM for sample image I will be $s(i) = [1.375; 2.25; 0.875; 0; 4.625]$. The five features defined below are derived from the 1-D matrix $s(i)$:

a. *Coarseness (COS)*: This is one of the fundamental properties of texture. A coarse texture is considered to have a high value of local uniformity in grey-level tones. Therefore, neighbouring pixel intensities are found almost similar, which subsequently infer the small difference between the grey-level tones of pixels and the average values of tones of the neighbouring pixels. The sum of the different terms which is calculated for all pixels in an image indicates the coarseness level of an image texture. This is defined as:

$$COS = \left[\epsilon + \sum_{i=0}^{G_h} p_i s(i) \right]^{-1}, \tag{6.47}$$

where G_h is the highest grey-tone value present in the image, ϵ is the small number to prevent COS becoming infinite and P_i is the probability of occurrence of grey-tone value i in an $N \times N$ image, given by:

$$p_i = \frac{N_i}{n^2}, \text{where } n = N - 2d. \tag{6.48}$$

Larger values of COS will represent areas where grey-tone differences are small, that is, of a coarse texture.

b. *Contrast (CON)*: An image is said to have good contrast if areas of different intensity levels are clearly visible. High contrast means that the intensity difference between neighbouring regions is large. It is calculated using:

$$CON = \left[\frac{1}{N_g(N_{g-1})} \sum_{i=0}^{G_h} \sum_{j=0}^{G_h} p_i p_j (i-j)^2 \right] \left[\frac{1}{n^2} \sum_{i=0}^{G_h} s(i) \right], \qquad (6.49)$$

where N_g indicates the number of grey values in the image; the CON represents the product of two terms; and the first term indicates the average value of weighted squared difference between the grey values of tones between the pixel pairs. The CON value shows a reflection of the dynamic range of the grey level, and the weighing factor is determined by the product of the probabilities of the two grey values of tones. The second represents the average value of difference between the grey tones of the pixel and the average grey-tone value in the neighbourhoods. If local variation in intensity is reported, then the value of the term is increased.

c. *Busyness (BUS)*: In busy texture there is rapid change in grey tone from one pixel to its neighbour. It is computed using:

$$BUS = \frac{\displaystyle\sum_{i=0}^{G_h} p_i s(i)}{\displaystyle\sum_{i=0}^{G_h} \sum_{j=0}^{G_h} (ip_i - jp_j)}, p_i \neq 0, p_j \neq 0. \qquad (6.50)$$

The numerator in the ratio indicates the rate of spatial change in intensity value, and the denominator represents the magnitude of difference between the grey values of tones.

d. *Complexity (COM)*: This metric indicates the content of visual information of the texture in an image. We can calculate ths value using:

$$COM = \left\{ \sum_{i=0}^{G_h} \sum_{j=0}^{G_h} \left[\frac{|i-j|}{(n^2(p_i + p_j))} \right] (p_i s(i) + p_j s(j)) \right\}, p_i \neq 0, p_j \neq 0 \qquad (6.51)$$

The COM value here indicates the sum of normalized values of differences between pixel intensity values, considered in pixel pairs. The weighing is computed for all the difference terms by using a probability-weighted function in the NGTDM that corresponds to the two intensity values.

e. *Texture strength (STR)*: Texture is referred to as strong when the primitives that comprise it are easily definable and clearly visible. It is calculated using:

$$STR = \frac{\displaystyle\sum_{i=0}^{G_h}\sum_{j=0}^{G_h}(p_i + p_j)(i - j)^2}{\displaystyle\in + \sum_{i=0}^{G_h} s(i)}, p_i \neq 0, p_j \neq 0. \qquad (6.52)$$

The numerator of the above ratio emphasizes the difference terms between intensity levels and the denominator refers to the size of texture primitives.

6.3.5 STATISTICAL FEATURE MATRIX

A statistical feature matrix (SFM) for texture analysis in [15] suggests that M_{sf} in the matrix has a dimension of $(L_r +1) \times (2L_c +1)$, in which (i, j) represents an element and d is referred to as a statistical feature of the image. The value of d is in the range $j - L_r$, i that indicates the spacing distance between the samples. For vectors $I = 0$, 1, 2, ..., L_r, $j = 0, 1, 2, ...,$ $2L_c$, the values of L_r, L_c are constants used for estimating the maximum value of inter-sample spacing distance [15]. There are four texture features: contrast, coarseness, roughness and periodicity, and these can be calculated using:

a. *Coarseness (COS)*: Measurement of coarseness is defined as:

$$COS = \frac{c}{\displaystyle\sum_{(i,j)\in N_r} DSS(i, j)/n}, \qquad (6.53)$$

where c is a normalizing factor, N_r is the set of displacement vectors defined as:

$$N_r = \{(i, j): |i|, |j| \leq r\}, \qquad (6.54)$$

and n is the number of elements in the set. The value of $r (= L_r = L_c)$ and c are arbitrarily chosen to be 4 and 100 respectively [15]. Further, if $\delta(dx, dy)$ is the inter-sampling distance, then the dissimilarity measure DSS is defined as:

$$DSS(\delta) = E\{|I(x, y) - I(x + dx, y + dy)|\}, \qquad (6.55)$$

where $E\{\cdot\}$ denotes the expectation operation. The denominator of Equation (6.53) will be low for a coarser image, giving a larger value of COS.

b. *Contrast (CON)*: The most important factor for the contrast of an image is the sharpness of edges which can be measured by:

$$CON = \left[\sum_{(i,j) \in N_r} con(i,j)/4 \right]^{\frac{1}{2}}, \tag{6.56}$$

where N_r is defined as in Equation (6.54) and $con(\delta)$ is given by:

$$con(\delta) = E\left\{ [I(x,y) - I(x+dx, y+dy)]^2 \right\}. \tag{6.57}$$

c. *Periodicity (PER)*: The measure of periodicity is defined as:

$$PER = \frac{\overline{M_{dss}} - M_{dss}(valley)}{\overline{M_{dss}}}, \tag{6.58}$$

where M_{dss} is defined as the dissimilarity matrix of the image whose *(i,j)* elements are the values of $DSS(\delta)$, $\overline{M_{dss}}$ is the mean of all elements in M_{dss}, and M_{dss} (valley) is the deepest valley in the matrix.

d. *Roughness (RGH)*: The measure of roughness of the image is given by:

$$RGH = \left(D_f^{(h)} + D_f^{(v)} \right)/2, \tag{6.59}$$

where $D_f^{(h)}$ and $D_f^{(v)}$ are the fractal dimensions in horizontal and vertical directions calculated using:

$$D_f = 3 - H \tag{6.60}$$

and H is the *(i, j + L_c)th* element of the dissimilarity matrix. The larger value of D_f indicates a rough image. In addition, an image with the same $D_f^{(h)}$ and $D_f^{(v)}$ is called isotropic; otherwise, it is called anisotropic.

6.3.6 Texture Energy Measures

Variations in intensities and texture are measured using a texture energy approach [16] for fixed-size windows in images. The measures are used in texture analysis [17], in which nine 7×7 convolution masks are utilized for measuring the texture energy. This is expressed as a vector in which each pixel of the image is analysed. We can compute the masks by using:

$$L7 \ (level) = [W] \tag{6.61a}$$

$$E7 \ (edge) = [-1 \ -4 \ -5 \ 0 \ 5 \ 4 \ 1] \tag{6.61b}$$

$$S7 \ (spot) = [-1 \ -2 \ 1 \ 4 \ 1 \ -2 \ -1], \tag{6.61c}$$

where $L7$ is a vector indicating centre weighted local average; $E7$ is used to detect the edges in the images; and spots are detected by $S7$. We can also use other masks of 3×3 or 5×5 that can produce convolution masks of size 3×3 or 5×5 respectively [16–18]. 2D convolution masks are obtained by computing the product of a pair of vectors.

For example, the mask $L7E7$ is computed by multiplying $L7$ and $E7$, as illustrated below:

$$\begin{bmatrix} 1 \\ 6 \\ 15 \\ 20 \\ 15 \\ 6 \\ 1 \end{bmatrix} \times \begin{bmatrix} -1 & -4 & -5 & 0 & 5 & 4 & 1 \end{bmatrix} = \begin{bmatrix} -1 & -4 & -5 & 0 & 5 & 4 & 1 \\ -6 & -24 & -30 & 0 & 30 & 24 & 6 \\ -15 & -60 & -75 & 0 & 75 & 60 & 15 \\ -20 & -80 & -100 & 0 & 100 & 80 & 20 \\ -15 & -60 & -75 & 0 & 75 & 60 & 15 \\ -6 & -24 & -30 & 0 & 30 & 24 & 6 \\ -1 & -4 & -5 & 0 & 5 & 4 & 1 \end{bmatrix} \dots$$

$$\tag{6.62}$$

The masks $L7L7$, $E7E7$, $S7S7$, $L7E7$, $E7L7$, $E7S7$, $S7E7$, $L7S7$, and $S7L7$ are computed, each of size 7×7. The masks are used to pre-process the images, and we obtain the nine corresponding filtered images using 9 masks. If $F_k[i, j]$ is the filtered image using the kth mask at pixel position $[i, j]$m then the texture energy map E_k of window size 15×15 is:

$$E_k[r,c] = \sum_{j=c-7}^{c+7} \sum_{i=r-7}^{r+7} \left| F_k[i,j] \right| \dots \tag{6.63}$$

Then, we calculate the average value of symmetric pairs, which are used to produce six maps. For example, $L7E7$ is used to measure the vertical edge gradient, and the horizontal edge gradient is measured by using $E7L7$. The content of edges in the image is computed with the help of maps $L7L7$, $E7E7$, $S7S7$, $L7E7/ E7L7$, $E7S7/ S7E7$, and $L7S7/ S7L7$, which result in a single vector having six attributes of texture.

6.3.7 Fractal Dimension Texture Analysis

Roughness is another important attribute which is used to measure the texture in images, and the fractional Brownian motion model is considered an important method of measuring the roughness of natural surfaces [12]. The fractal dimension is used to represent the fractal surface in the images. Texture analysis using a dimension approach utilizes a number of texture features having multiple resolution, and a few of them can summarized as:

a. Determine $I^{(m)}, I^{(m-1)},\ldots\ldots,I^{(m-n+1)}$ as n resolution images (where $m = log_2 M$) using:

$$I^{(i)}(x,y) = \frac{\left[I^{(i+1)}(2x,2y) + I^{(i+1)}(2x+1,2y) + I^{(i+1)}(2x,2y+1) + I^{(i+1)}(2x+1,2y+1)\right]}{4} \ldots\ldots,$$

(6.64)

where $I^{(i)}(x,y)$ is the image at resolution level i with $0 \le i \le m$ and $0 \le x, y \le 2^i$.

b. Determine H: Given an $M \times M$ image I, the intensity difference vector is defined as:

$$IDV = [id(1), id(2),\ldots\ldots\ldots\ldots id(s)], \tag{6.65}$$

where s is the maximum possible scale and $id(k)$ is the average of the absolute intensity difference of all pixel pairs with horizontal or vertical distance k, given by:

$$id(k) = \frac{\sum\limits_{x=0}^{M-1}\sum\limits_{y=0}^{M-k-1}|I(x,y) - I(x,y+k)| + \sum\limits_{x=0}^{M-k-1}\sum\limits_{y=0}^{M-1}|I(x,y) - I(x+k,y)|}{2M(M-k-1)}. \tag{6.66}$$

The least square regression is used to obtain H value by determining the slope of the curve of $id(k)$ with respect to k in log-log scales.

c. Find the fractal dimension as per Equation (6.60).
d. Collect the fractal dimensions of images having different resolutions that correspond to fractal feature set of multi-resolution, as:

$$MF = \left(H^{(m)}, H^{(m-1)},\ldots\ldots,H^{(m-n+1)}\right), \tag{6.67}$$

where $M = 2^m$, denotes image size of the original image, $H^{(k)}$ is used to denote H parameter that can be computed from $I^{(k)}$, and number of resolutions is denoted by n. We have extracted features of four different resolutions for $k = 1$, 2, 3, 4.

6.3.8 SPECTRAL MEASURES OF TEXTURE

Texture discrimination and characterization are used in texture analysis with the help of the Fourier spectrum, and the features are referred to as spectrum-based texture features [8, 11, 12, 19–21]. Periodic and non-periodic texture features or patterns are used as spectral texture features that help in discriminating images. The difference terms can be easily quantized if we can get feature sets differently using spectral analysis between periodic patterns [18]. Let F(u, v) be the Discrete Fourier Transform (DFT) of image I(x, y), then the sample power spectrum is computed using:

$$\varphi(u,v) = F(u,v)F^*(u,v) = \left| F(u,v) \right|^2, \tag{6.68}$$

where φ indicates the sample power spectrum and * is used to represent the complex conjugate. Higher values of $|F|^2$ are reported for coarse texture values, which are concentrated around the origin, and the larger spread out is observed for fine texture values of the images. When there are many edges and lines in a certain direction θ, then higher values of $|F|^2$ concentrated around a perpendicular direction $\theta + \pi/2$ produce textures, and a homogeneous texture will have a value of $|F|^2$ as directional [12]. The spectrum in polar coordinates using spectrum features is used to produce a function S(r, θ), where S denotes the spectrum function, and r and θ are two coordinate values in the spectral coordinate system. For each direction θ, S(r, θ) may be chosen as 1D function $S_\theta(r)$. In a similar manner, for each frequency r, $S_r(\theta)$ again becomes a 1D function and the analysis of $S_\theta(r)$ for a fixed value of θ produces the spectrum behaviour along a radial direction from the origin. The analysis of $S_r(\theta)$ for a fixed value of r produces a spectrum behaviour along a circle which is centred around the origin [8].

The integration as a sum of discrete variables is used as the function of feature estimation, as [8, 16]:

$$S(r) = \sum_{\theta=0}^{\pi} S_\theta(r) \tag{6.69}$$

$$S(\theta) = \sum_{r=1}^{R_0} S_r(\theta), \tag{6.70}$$

where R_0 is the radius of the circle centred at the origin. By varying the values of (r, θ), two 1D functions, S(r) and S(θ), are generated, which constitute a spectral energy description of the region of interest.

6.3.9 RUN-LENGTH TEXTURE FEATURES

Texture features are also determined using the run-length method [22–25] by classi-fying the texture values, which is considered an important method for the analysis of biomedical images. A run in the method is the sequence here that scans the direction of the pixels with identical values in the image; and the length indicates the number of pixels in the run. Therefore, the run-length features are used to encode the textural information corresponding to the number of times each grey level appears as single as well as in the form of pairs. For an image of size 4×4, the image $I(m, n)$ can be expressed as:

$$I(m,n) = \begin{bmatrix} 0 & 2 & 0 & 0 \\ 1 & 2 & 2 & 2 \\ 1 & 2 & 3 & 1 \\ 0 & 1 & 2 & 3 \end{bmatrix}. \tag{6.71}$$

The image $I(m, n)$ has four grey levels (0–3). The corresponding run-length matrices for various orientations and distance $d = 1$ are shown below:

$$I_{RL}(0^0) = \begin{bmatrix} 2 & 1 & 0 & 0 \\ 4 & 0 & 0 & 0 \\ 3 & 0 & 1 & 0 \\ 2 & 0 & 0 & 0 \end{bmatrix} \tag{6.72}$$

$$I_{RL}(90^0) = \begin{bmatrix} 4 & 0 & 0 & 0 \\ 2 & 1 & 0 & 0 \\ 3 & 0 & 1 & 0 \\ 2 & 0 & 0 & 0 \end{bmatrix} \tag{6.73}$$

$$I_{RL}(45^0) = \begin{bmatrix} 4 & 0 & 0 & 0 \\ 4 & 0 & 0 & 0 \\ 3 & 1 & 0 & 0 \\ 2 & 0 & 0 & 0 \end{bmatrix} \tag{6.74}$$

$$I_{RL}(135^0) = \begin{bmatrix} 4 & 0 & 0 & 0 \\ 2 & 1 & 0 & 0 \\ 2 & 2 & 1 & 0 \\ 0 & 1 & 0 & 0 \end{bmatrix}. \tag{6.75}$$

We obtain the texture features for each value of d *considering all* the four orientations, and the values are averaged so that the texture features become rotation invariant, as required in GLCM texture features. Suppose the $p(i, j)$ is the $(i, j)^{th}$ entry for a run-length matrix; N_g indicates grey levels in the image; N_r denotes the number of different run lengths; and p is the number of points in the image. For this consideration, 11 texture features are extracted using run-length matrices [22–25]:

a. *Short run emphasis [SRE]*: This feature increases when the short run dominates. It is defined as:

$$SRE = \frac{\sum_{i=1}^{N_g} \sum_{j=1}^{N_r} \left(p(i, j)/j^2 \right)}{\sum_{i=1}^{N_g} \sum_{j=1}^{N_r} p(i, j)}. \tag{6.76}$$

The denominator of Equation (6.76) is the total number of run lengths in the matrix. SRE function emphasizes small run lengths due to division by j^2.

b. *Long run emphasis [LRE]*: This feature increases when the long run dominates. It is computed using:

$$LRE = \frac{\sum_{i=1}^{N_g} \sum_{j=1}^{N_r} \left(p(i, j)j^2 \right)}{\sum_{i=1}^{N_g} \sum_{j=1}^{N_r} p(i, j)}. \tag{6.77}$$

This function multiplies each run-length value by the length of the run squared. Hence, it emphasizes long runs.

c. *Grey-level non-uniformity [GLNU]*: It measures the grey-level non-uniformity of the image; that is, it is lower when runs are equally distributed throughout the grey levels. It is defined by:

$$GLNU = \frac{\sum_{i=1}^{N_g} \left(\sum_{j=1}^{N_r} p(i, j) \right)^2}{\sum_{i=1}^{N_g} \sum_{j=1}^{N_r} p(i, j)}. \tag{6.78}$$

d. *Run-length non-uniformity [RLNU]*: It measures the non-uniformity of run lengths; that is, it is lower when runs are equally distributed throughout the lengths. It is computed by using:

$$RLNU = \frac{\sum\limits_{j=1}^{N_g}\left(\sum\limits_{i=1}^{N_r} p(i,j)\right)^2}{\sum\limits_{i=1}^{N_g}\sum\limits_{j=1}^{N_r} p(i,j)}. \tag{6.79}$$

e. *Run percentage [RPC]*: It is the ratio of the total number of runs to the total number of possible runs if all runs had length one. Its value is higher for a linear image. It is defined as:

$$RPC = \frac{\sum\limits_{i=1}^{N_g}\sum\limits_{j=1}^{N_r} p(i,j)}{p}. \tag{6.80}$$

f. *Low grey-level run emphasis [LGRE]*: This feature makes use of the distribution of grey levels for runs. It increases when the texture is dominated by many runs of low grey value. It is defined as:

$$LGRE = \frac{\sum\limits_{i=1}^{N_g}\sum\limits_{j=1}^{N_r}\left(p(i,j)/i^2\right)}{\sum\limits_{i=1}^{N_g}\sum\limits_{j=1}^{N_r} p(i,j)}. \tag{6.81}$$

g. *High grey-level run emphasis [HGRE]*: This feature also makes use of the distribution of grey levels for runs. It increases when the texture is dominated by many runs of high grey value. It is defined as:

$$HGRE = \frac{\sum\limits_{i=1}^{N_g}\sum\limits_{j=1}^{N_r}\left(p(i,j)i^2\right)}{\sum\limits_{i=1}^{N_g}\sum\limits_{j=1}^{N_r} p(i,j)}. \tag{6.82}$$

The remaining four features proposed in [24] emphasize the joint distribution properties of the run lengths and grey levels instead of the individual ones separately. They
are defined below:

a. *Short-run low grey-level emphasis [SRLGE]*: This feature combines SRE and
   LGRE. It will increase when the texture is dominated by many short runs of low
   grey value. It is defined as:

$$SRLGE = \frac{\sum\limits_{i=1}^{N_g} \sum\limits_{j=1}^{N_r} \left(p(i,j)/i^2 j^2 \right)}{\sum\limits_{i=1}^{N_g} \sum\limits_{j=1}^{N_r} p(i,j)}. \tag{6.83}$$

b. *Short-run high grey-level emphasis [SRHGE]*: This feature combines SRE and
   HGRE. It will increase when the texture is dominated by many short runs of
   high grey value. It is defined as:

$$SRHGE = \frac{\sum\limits_{i=1}^{N_g} \sum\limits_{j=1}^{N_r} \left(p(i,j)i^2 \right)/j^2}{\sum\limits_{i=1}^{N_g} \sum\limits_{j=1}^{N_r} p(i,j)}. \tag{6.84}$$

c. *Long-run high grey-level emphasis [LRHGE]*: This feature is complementary
   to SRLGE. It increases with a combination of long, high grey value runs. It is
   computed using:

$$LRHGE = \frac{\sum\limits_{i=1}^{N_g} \sum\limits_{j=1}^{N_r} \left(p(i,j)i^2 j^2 \right)}{\sum\limits_{i=1}^{N_g} \sum\limits_{j=1}^{N_r} p(i,j)}. \tag{6.85}$$

d. *Long-run low grey-level emphasis [LRLGE]*: This feature is complementary to
   SRHGE. It increases when the texture dominated by long runs that have low
   grey levels. It is defined by:

$$LRLGE \frac{\sum\limits_{i=1}^{N_g} \sum\limits_{j=1}^{N_r} \left(p(i,j)i^2 \right)/j^2}{\sum\limits_{i=1}^{N_g} \sum\limits_{j=1}^{N_r} p(i,j)}. \tag{6.86}$$

6.4   SHAPE FEATURE EXTRACTION

The shape and size of images are of good significance in medical image analysis and its applications, which are extracted from suitable ROIs in which diagnostic content is present in the images. For example, for breast cancer detection and analysis using ultrasound images, tumour detection is estimated with the help of size and shape features differentiating malignant and benign masses in the images. We know that benign masses have regular shapes and malignant tissues are indicated by irregular shapes that are reflected by shape and size features. Also, in many cases it has been seen that nodules with a perimeter of more than 3 cm are usually malignant. In this study, the following shape and size features are extracted:

6.4.1   REGION PROPERTIES

Three simple regional features, namely area, perimeter and compactness, are commonly used for the quantification of object shape. These regional properties are based on grey-level intensities [8]. The area of a region can be defined as the number of pixels in the region. The second measure in this category is perimeter. For a region in a 2D image, the parameter can be computed after the identification of its boundary pixels.

Let us suppose that the boundary of a region comprises an ordered sequence of pixels defined in the x-y coordinate system. The pixels are connected with either four or eight connectivity. The distance between two consecutive pixels is 1 or $\sqrt{2}$ units if they are four or eight connected respectively. The perimeter of a 2D shape is then determined by calculating the total distance around the shape. The third measure, compactness, is a measure of circularity defined by:

$$Compactness = \frac{(Perimeter)^2}{Area}. \tag{6.87}$$

6.4.2   MOMENT INVARIANTS

In pattern recognition and medical diagnosis methods, moment invariant features are used that convey very rich information about the patterns in the images. Each moment coefficient and its invariant carries a proper value of information which is extracted from the medical image [9]. Considering $f(x, y)$ as an original image, the 2D moment of order $(p+q)$ [8] can be calculated by:

$$m_{pq} = \sum_x \sum_y x^p y^q f(x,y), \text{for } p,q = 0,1,2,\ldots\ldots, \tag{6.88}$$

where the summations are over the values of the spatial coordinates x and y spanning the image. The corresponding central moment is defined as:

$$\mu_{pq} = \sum_x \sum_y (x - \bar{x})^p (y - \bar{y})^q f(x,y), \tag{6.89}$$

where $\bar{x} = \dfrac{m_{10}}{m_{00}}$ and $\bar{y} = \dfrac{m_{01}}{m_{00}}$. The normalized central moment of order $(p+q)$ is defined as:

$$\eta_{pq} = \frac{\mu_{pq}}{\mu_{00}^{\gamma}}, \text{for } p,q = 0, 1, 2, \ldots \ldots , \tag{6.90}$$

where

$$\gamma = \frac{p+q}{2} + 1, \text{for p+q=2,3,\ldots \ldots} \tag{6.91}$$

The size, orientation and position of the objects play important role in pattern analysis [26]. There are seven invariant moments which do not change irrespective of translation, scaling, mirroring and rotation, as reported in Hu [27]. The moments are:

$$\varphi_1 = \eta_{20} + \eta_{02} \tag{6.92}$$

$$\varphi_2 = \left(\eta_{20} - \eta_{02}\right)^2 + 4\eta_{11}^2 \tag{6.93}$$

$$\varphi_3 = \left(\eta_{30} - 3\eta_{12}\right)^2 + \left(\eta_{03} - 3\eta_{21}\right)^2 \tag{6.94}$$

$$\varphi_4 = \left(\eta_{30} + \eta_{12}\right)^2 + \left(\eta_{03} + \eta_{21}\right)^2 \tag{6.95}$$

$$\begin{aligned}\varphi_5 &= \left(\eta_{30} - 3\eta_{12}\right)\left(\eta_{30} + \eta_{12}\right)\left[\left(\eta_{30} + \eta_{12}\right)^2 - 3\left(\eta_{21} + \eta_{03}\right)^2\right] \\ &+ \left(\eta_{03} - 3\eta_{21}\right)\left(\eta_{03} + \eta_{21}\right)\left[\left(\eta_{03} + \eta_{21}\right)^2 - 3\left(\eta_{12} + \eta_{30}\right)^2\right]\end{aligned} \tag{6.96}$$

$$\begin{aligned}\varphi_6 &= \left(\eta_{20} - \eta_{02}\right)\left[\left(\eta_{30} + \eta_{12}\right)^2 - \left(\eta_{21} + \eta_{03}\right)^2\right] \\ &+ 4\eta_{11}\left(\eta_{30} + \eta_{12}\right)\left(\eta_{03} + \eta_{21}\right)\end{aligned} \tag{6.97}$$

$$\begin{aligned}\varphi_7 &= \left(3\eta_{21} - \eta_{03}\right)\left(\eta_{30} + \eta_{12}\right)\left[\left(\eta_{30} + \eta_{12}\right)^2 - 3\left(\eta_{21} + \eta_{03}\right)^2\right] \\ &+ \left(\eta_{30} - 3\eta_{12}\right)\left(\eta_{21} + \eta_{03}\right)\left[\left(\eta_{03} + \eta_{21}\right)^2 - 3\left(\eta_{30} + \eta_{12}\right)^2\right].\end{aligned} \tag{6.98}$$

6.5   FEATURE NORMALIZATION

Feature extraction is followed by feature normalization, which acts as a pre-processing technique to feature selection. The features are normalized before the most suitable features are selected for the applications. The features obtained from a number of real-time images may be of different sources utilizing different feature extraction algorithms, and thus it becomes necessary to normalize the feature data before we actually select the useful features. In the process of data normalization, we can normalize the various dynamic ranges of the data. The Euclidean distance is generally used for normalizing the data over a dynamic range of feature data. A large dynamic range is converted into a suitable and useful small range of feature data using normalization techniques. So, some similarity measures are used in the normalization process [28]. If the small-range and most suitable data is subjected to further stages such as classification, then the proper classified outcomes result from the real-time patterns present in the images.

When applying normalization methods for features, the choice of the method and range is very important so that the structure of the data becomes appropriate, and multivariate analysis is useful for image and pattern analysis [28]. We have examined a few important case studies on normalization techniques in [29–33], and this study suggests that there is no robust or general purpose dataset, normalization method or range of data values [31].

6.5.1   BRIEF OVERVIEW OF FEATURE NORMALIZATION TECHNIQUES

Suppose x_i and $\hat{x}_i$ are the original and the normalized features respectively and the feature set contains "N" values. A summary of the different normalization methods in the study is as follows:

a. *Z – Score normalization*: This method uses unit variance and zero mean, which are assigned to the feature set as a process of normalization [29]. This is considered a linear method in which the initial values of mean ($\bar{x}$) and the standard deviation (σ) are computed for a specific feature with the help of:

$$\bar{x} = \frac{1}{N} \sum_{i=1}^{N} x_i \tag{6.99}$$

$$\sigma^2 = \frac{1}{N-1} \sum_{i=1}^{N} (x_i - \bar{x})^2. \tag{6.100}$$

The feature after normalized feature is:

$$\hat{x}_i = \frac{x_i - \bar{x}}{\sigma}, i = 1, 2 \ldots \ldots N. \tag{6.101}$$

b. *Min–Max normalization*: A linear function is used to transform the features by mapping the values using an attribute x_i from the range $[\min(x_i), \max(x_i)]$ to a new range $[\min x_{new}, \max x_{new}]$. The features after normalization are:

$$\hat{x}_i = \frac{x_i - \min(x_i)}{\max(x_i) - \min(x_i)}(\max x_{new} - \min x_{new}) + \min x_{new}. \qquad (6.102)$$

This method has the ability to preserve the inherent relationships among the original data values [30]. The values in the method were chosen as $\max x_{new} = 1$, $\min x_{new} = -1$.

c. *Linear scaling to unit range*: A linear transformation is used to bring the feature data in range [0, 1]. For a lower bound $\min(x_i)$ and upper bound $\max(x_i)$ of an attribute x_i, the data after normalization is:

$$\hat{x}_i = \frac{x_i - \min(x_i)}{\max(x_i) - \min(x_i)}. \qquad (6.103)$$

Linear scaling for converting into the unit range is an example of min-max normalization having $\max x_{new} = 1$ and $\min x_{new} = 0$.

d. *Softmax scaling*: The scaling, linear and non-linear methods do not normalize the values evenly distributed around the mean [9]. In this case, other types of methods having non-linear functions such as exponential, logarithmic, sigmoid and so on are used for mapping the data values into desired ranges or intervals. As an example, softmax scaling is used to squash the data values in the range [0, 1]. The features after normalization become:

$$\hat{x}_i = \frac{1}{1 + e^{-y}}, \qquad (6.104)$$

where $y = \dfrac{x_i - \bar{x}}{r\sigma}$ and r are parameters that can be set by the user. For smaller

values of y values of x_i closer to the mean, y is produced using the linear function approximately. Other values of x and y are squashed exponentially.

LEARNING OUTCOME

Students, after completion of this chapter, will be able to explain

- Feature extraction methods
- Importance of feature normalization

REFERENCES

1. Popli, M. B. (2002). Pictorial essay: Sonographic differentiation of solid breast lesions. *Indian Journal of Radiology and Imaging, 12*, 275–279.

2. Calas, M. J. G., Koch, H. A., & Dutra, M. V. P. (2007). Breast ultrasound: Evaluation of echographic criteria for differentiation of breast lesions. *Radiologia Brasileira, 40*, 1–7.

3. American College of Radiology. (2003). *BI-RADS-US Lexicon Classification*. www. acr.org/Clinical-Resources/Reporting-and-Data-Systems/Bi-Rads

4. Raza, Sughra, Goldkamp, Allison, L., Chikarmane, Sona A., & Birdwell, Robyn L. (2010). US of breast masses categorized as BI-RADS 3, 4, and 5: Pictorial review of factors influencing clinical management. *Radiographics, 30*, 1199–1213.

5. Haralick, R. M., Shanmugam, K., & Dinstein, I. (1973). Textural features for image classification. *IEEE Transactions on Systems, Man & Cybernetics*, SMC-6, 610–621.

6. Tuceryan, M., & Jain, A. K. (1998). Texture analysis. In C. H. Chen, L. F. Pau, & P. S. P. Wang (Eds.), *The handbook of pattern recognition and computer vision* (2nd ed.) (pp. 207–248). World Scientific Publishing.

7. Srinivasan, G. N., & Shobha, G. (2008). Statistical texture analysis. *Proceedings of World Academy of Science, Engineering and Technology, 36*, 1264–1269.

8. Gonzalez, R. C., & Woods, R. E. (2010). *Digital image processing using MATLAB* (2nd ed.). Pearson Prentice Hall.

9. Theodoridis, S., & Koutroumbas, K. (2009). *Pattern recognition* (4th ed.). Elsevier.

10. Haralick, R. M. (1979). Statistical and structural approaches to texture. *Proceedings IEEE, 67*, 786–804.

11. Weszka, J. S., Dyer, C. R., & Rosenfeld, A. (1976). A comparative study of texture measures for terrain classification. *IEEE Transactions on Systems, Man and Cybernetics*, SMC-6, 269–285.

12. Wu, C. M., Chen, Y. C., & Hsieh, K. S. (1992). Texture features for classification of ultrasonic liver images. *IEEE Transactions on Medical Imaging, 11*, 141–152, 1992.

13. Amadasun, M., & King, R. (1989). Texture features corresponding to textural properties. *IEEE Transactions on Systems, Man and Cybernetics, 19*, 1264–1274.

14. Stoitsi, John, Golemati, Spyretta, & Nikita, Konstantina S. (2006). A modular software system to assist interpretation of medical images – application to vascular ultrasound images. *IEEE Transactions on Instrumentation and Measurement, 55*, 1944–1952.

15. Wu, Chung-Ming, & Chen, Yung-Chang. (1992). Statistical feature matrix for texture analysis. *CVGIP: Graphical Models and Image Processing, 54*, 407–419.

16. Laws, Kenneth I. (1980). Rapid texture identification. *Image Processing for Missile Guidance, 238*, 376–380.

17. Xie, X., & Mirmehdi, M. (2008). A galaxy of texture features. In M. Mirmehdi, X. Xie, & J. Suri (Eds.), *Handbook of texture analysis* (pp. 347–406). Imperial College Press.

18. Shapiro, Linda G., & Stockman, George C. (2000). *Texture* (ch. 7). Computer Vision. https://courses.cs.washington.edu/courses/cse576.

19. Dyer, Charles R., & Rosenfeld, Azriel. (1976). Fourier texture features: Suppression of aperture effects. *IEEE Transactions on Systems, Man and Cybernetics, 6*, 703–705.

20. Stromberg, William D., & Farr, Tom G. (1986). A Fourier based textural feature extraction procedure. *IEEE Transactions on Geoscience and Remote Sensing* (Vol. GE-24). IEEE.

21. Feng Zhou, Ju-Fu Feng, & Shi, Qing-yun. (2001). Texture feature based on local Fourier transform. *Proceedings of International Conference on Image Processing, 2*, 610–613.

22. Galloway, Mary M. (1975). Texture analysis using grey level run lengths. *Computer Graphics and Image Processing, 4*, 172–179.
23. Chu, A., Sehgal, C. M., & Greenleaf, J. F. (1990). Use of grey value distribution of run lengths for texture analysis. *Pattern Recognition Letters, 11*, 415–420.
24. Dasarathy, Belur V., & Holder, Edwin B. (1991). Image characterizations based on joint grey level run length distributions. *Pattern Recognition Letters, 12*, 497–502.
25 Tang, Xiaoou (1998). *Texture information in run length matrices. IEEE Transactions on Image Processing, 7*, 1602–1609.
26. Mercimek, Muharrem, Gulez, Kayhan, & Mumcu, Tarik Veli. (2005). Real object recognition using moment invariants. *Sadhana, 30*, 765–775.
27. Hu, Ming-Kuei. (1962). Visual pattern recognition by moment invariants. *IRE Transactions on Information Theory, 8*, 179–187.
28. Salama, M. A., Hassanien, A. E., & Fahmy, A. A. (2010). Reducing the influence of normalization on data classification. *2010 International Conference on Computer Information Systems and Industrial Management Applications (CISIM)*, 609–613.
29. Aksoy, S., & Haralick, R. (2000). Feature normalization and likelihood-based similarity measures for image retrieval. *Pattern Recognition Letters*, Special Issue on Image and Video Retrieval.
30. Manikandan, G., Sairam, N., Sharmili, S., & Venkatakrishnan, S. (2013). Achieving privacy in data mining using normalization. *Indian Journal of Science and Technology, 6*, 4268–4272.
31. Patel, Vaishali R., & Mehta, Rupa G. (2011). Impact of outlier removal and normalization approach in modified k-means clustering algorithm. *International Journal of Computer Science Issues, 8*, 331–336.
32. Saranya, C., & Manikandan, G. (2013). A study on normalization techniques for privacy preserving data mining. *International Journal of Engineering and Technology, 5*, 2701–2704.
33. Jayalakshmi, T., & Santhakumaran, A. (2011). Statistical normalization and back propagation for classification. *International Journal of Computer Theory and Engineering, 3*, 89–93.

7 Introduction to Machine Learning

LEARNING OBJECTIVES

This chapter aims to cover:

- Overview and classification of machine learning (ML)
- Steps of implementation of ML techniques
- Testing, training and validation processes involved in ML methods
- Major ML techniques and their performance metrics

This chapter highlights an overview of machine learning methods as machine learning plays a most important role in feature extraction and interpretation of medical images. Some training is required to interpret a huge amount of image-related data, which is achieved by using a suitable machine learning technique.

7.1 INTRODUCTION: WHAT IS MACHINE LEARNING?

In any image processing task, the role of machine learning is significant because machine learning methods only assist in interpreting a huge amount of image data through suitable training or the learning process. The term "machine learning" was introduced by an American researcher, Arthur Samuel, as a tool that could empower the computers with capabilities to learn data explicitly. The machine learning term was coined in 1959 [1]. Later, in 1997, another researcher, Tom Mitchell [2], explained machine learning as a relational method in which the machine is programmed to perform some work/task "T" with a specified performance measure "P," and by performing the task multiple times, the machine gains experience "E" which improves the performance of the system. Then, as the system proceeds further, it gains more experience and the output performance becomes more precise.

To understand the term machine learning in a more simplified manner, let us consider the example of person trying to throw a ball into a basket. On the first attempt he misses the basket, so he tries again and this time he improves the shot with his past experience and throws it closer to the basket. After many unsuccessful attempts, the person make the ball go into the basket, and in this way, he is learning how to make a perfect shot into the basket. In the same way, a machine is allowed to learn with

DOI: 10.1201/9781003097808-7

past experience to improve the performance of a specified task with the help of a programme or algorithm. This process of improving the performance of a system using past system experience with the help of an algorithm is called machine learning.

Definition: Machine learning can be defined as the subset or a part of artificial intelligence (AI) which mainly focuses on designing various models of a system on the basis of data. The designed system is able to learn and also make predictions based on some experience that is the "data."

Before getting started with machine learning, let us take a glance at some of the important terminologies used in it.

SOME TERMINOLOGY OF MACHINE LEARNING

- **Model**: In machine learning, a model is used to represent real-world processing mathematically. This is also known as the "hypothesis." A model is built up by using any machine learning algorithm and a dataset.
- **Feature**: Any property or parameter of a dataset which can be measured in any scale can be a called a feature.
- **Feature Vector**: This is a set of various numeric features. It is used as an input to the machine learning model for training, testing and validation purposes.
- **Training**: This is a process in which an algorithm finds some pattern in the input data, which is known as training data, and accordingly trains the machine learning model to provide the expected results.
- **Prediction**: A machine learning model is designed to make predictions on the basis of a dataset when fed with an input to provide an output.
- **Target (Label)**: The value which has to be predicted by the machine learning model is called the target or label.
- **Overfitting**: When a machine learning model is trained by a massive amount of data, then it tends to learn from inaccurate data entries and noises. At this point the model fails to produce the accurate and desired output. This is due to overfitting.
- **Underfitting**: When a machine learning model is trained by a small amount of data and is not able to find a pattern in the input data. Then the accuracy of the machine learning model is hindered. This is due to underfitting.

7.2   CLASSIFICATION OF MACHINE LEARNING (ML) METHODS

There are a number of machine learning methods available in the literature as ML methods are computation algorithms for training data. The methods are categorized on the basis of some criteria. This section discusses the major categories of ML methods broadly used in medical image processing and its applications. The classification of ML techniques is as follows:

1. **Supervised learning:** In this type of ML method, the labelled input and output are always provided before the learning is applied. The values of different parameters or attributes are adjusted by training in such a manner that the desired response or output is obtained. The system later predicts the correct

response for the new object or new example that comes under the same class or string in which the training was initially applied to the input data. Such a type of learning is called supervised learning. Let us take an example of a teacher and a class. The teacher is telling the students about the difference between an apple and a mango, so for doing so she needs to tell them some difference in the property of an apple and a mango like the colour of a mango is yellow and of an apple is red. And the apple when cut is white inside whereas the mango is not. By knowing these basic differences, students can now always separate out apples and mangos for all possible cases after learning the basic appearance difference between the two fruits.

2. **Unsupervised learning:** In this type of learning the system learns from example data only and not any related response. This leads the algorithm to make assumptions on its own and determine the response and the data pattern on its own. This type of machine learning technique does not only restrict the data features to the conventional class or patterns but also restructures the data, which allows it to define new key features and classifications for the output data. This offers a better understanding of example data and provides useful new features for the supervised machine learning algorithm. This is similar to the method that humans generally use to classify different day-to-day objects and things by visual inspection, weight, colour, material and degree of similarity and so on.

3. **Reinforcement learning:** In this type of learning the presentation of example data is similar to unsupervised learning where no response is provided to the system. But the algorithm is provided with feedback by the user according to the understanding of the system and the proposed solution by the algorithm. This type of learning is similar to learning by one's own mistake, or also called the trial-and-error method in general. The type of algorithm that uses the aid of feedback to check the correctness of the proposed response for a given example comes under the category of reinforcement learning. In this type of algorithm, the system is made to take a decision and learn from its own mistakes if the feedback shows a negative response towards its solution.

4. **Semi-supervised learning:** In this type of learning the algorithm is given with all the possible example data, but the output data is not given for every case of input and the algorithm is allowed to predict the output for the corresponding input example data according to the given trend of responses given for some of the examples, and is provided with feedback to the response generated by the algorithm for whether it is correct or not. Negative feedback implies that the solution implemented by the algorithm is wrong and the system starts afresh for the calculation of the outcome of the input data by keeping in mind the old wrong responses.

7.3   STEPS IN IMPLEMENTATION OF MACHINE LEARNING

For complex tasks, machine learning can accomplish a lot. However, in order to simplify the method, a simple scenario is used to clarify the important aspects. We will

1. Gathering the data
2. Preparing the data
3. Choosing the model
4. Training
5. Evaluation
6. Hyper-parameter tuning
7. Prediction

FIGURE 7.1 Different steps of machine learning.

use an example of a simple model to show the importance and purpose of each move. This model would be responsible for differentiating between an apple and mango. Figure 7.1 shows seven major steps in the implementation of machine learning. AI's opportunities are vast, as it is rapidly becoming an essential component of a multitude of fields such as medicine, online business, finance and so on. Today, we will characterize AI as a system and understand the steps taken to get from its emergence to its practical implementation.

STEP 1: GATHERING DATA

The first step in designing our machine learning model will be to collect relevant data that can be used to distinguish between the two fruits. A variety of factors can be used to determine whether a fruit is an apple or a mango. For the sake of convenience, we will just look at two aspects that our model will employ in order to function. The colour of the fruit is the first unique feature, preceded by the shape of the fruit. We believe that by using these features, our model will be able to distinguish between the two fruits.

Colour	Shape	Apple or Mango
Red	Round	Apple
Yellow	Oval	Mango

The data for our two chosen features should be gathered by a device. For example, a spectrometer could be used to gather information on colouring, and images of organic products could be used to gather shape data, so they can be treated as 2D figures. To gain knowledge and understanding, we would continue to recover as many different types of apples and mangos as we could.

The very first step in the machine learning process is to obtain data. Missteps like picking the incorrect features or focusing on a small number of variations of entries for the dataset will make the model useless. That is why it is important to take the required precautions when collecting data, as mistakes made at this point will only escalate as we move to the later stages.

STEP 2: PREPARING THE DATA

When we have gathered details for the two highlights, separating the bits of knowledge into two parts is another important aspect of information preparation. The larger portion (80%) will be used to prepare the model, while the smaller portion (20%) will be used for evaluation purposes. This is crucial because whoever uses the same measures of information for both evaluation and assessment does not provide a fair assessment of the model's performance in real-world scenarios. Apart from the broken information, further improvements are made to the informational indexes. This may include removing duplicate passages, discarding inaccurate readings and so on. Solid and consistent data for your model will help it enhance its efficiency. It will help reduce the model's weak points, resulting in greater precision in expectations. As a result, it is a good idea to think about and audit your informational indexes so that they can be designed to produce stronger and more significant results.

STEP 3: CHOOSING A MODEL

After data is developed and prepared properly, the suitable model to be used is chosen for the application where machine learning will be applied. Various types of models exist for a number of applications used by numerous researchers based on the need and training attributes. The purpose of using ML, attributes to be used in training, dimension of data and so on play an important role when choosing the ML technique for the relevant applications.

For the purposes of our model, a simple direct relapse model is suitable for distinguishing between organic and non-organic products. The type of organic product would be our dependent variable, while the shade of the foods grown from the field of natural products would be the two measures or autonomous variables in this case.

The product choice was truly evident in our model. In more unpredictable cases, we must make a choice that aligns with our desired outcome. There are three different types of AI models that can be investigated. Controlled learning models are the most common classification. We refine the actual model until our yield reaches the optimal level of exactness in such models since the outcome is known. A good example of managed learning is the straight relapse model we used for our natural product model. The following classification, unaided learning, is used if the outcome is ambiguous and we need to make arrangements.

K-means and a priori approximation are examples of unaided instruction. Help learning is the third category. It is about finding out how to make better decisions by trial and error. These are most commonly used in professional settings. Its model is the Markov's choice interaction.

STEP 4: TRAINING

The planning of the model is at the heart of the AI interaction. At this stage, the majority of the "learning" has been completed. Here, we use the informational index that was circulated for preparation to demonstrate our model's ability to distinguish between the two natural products. If we think of our model in numerical terms, the data sources, such as our two highlights, would have coefficients. The tones of highlights are the names given to these coefficients. A clear or y-catch will be included as well. This is referred to as the model's tendency. Experimentation is the only way to determine their attributes. At first, we assign them arbitrary attributes and provide inputs. The actual yield is compared to the true yield, and the thing that matters is restricted by experimenting with different load and predisposition estimations. Various sections from our planning informational set are used to continue the emphases until the model is complete. Preparing can be extremely satisfying if the model succeeds in its task. It's almost the same as when a child learns to ride a bike. They may fall a few times at first, but they will eventually gain a better understanding of the interaction and be able to adapt to different situations when riding a bicycle.

STEP 5: EVALUATION

Once the data is prepared and the model is chosen and developed for an application, we need to test the model for the real-time application. The testing can be done in order to validate the capability of the information creation and evaluation. The testing process enables to model for better classifying and interpreting the data intended for an application. For example, if the model is expected to differentiate between two fruits like a mango and an apple, it must be able to do so using appropriate attributes. Regardless, the model should be capable of extrapolating the data and determining if the organic product is an apple or a mango through its preparation.

When it comes to business applications, evaluation has proven to be extremely important. Knowledge researchers may use assessment to see whether the goals they set for themselves were fulfilled or not. If the results aren't promising, the earlier progress should be revisited in order to identify and correct the underlying cause of the model's poor performance. If the evaluation isn't completed correctly, the model will not be able to fulfil the model's ideal business reason. This may mean that the company that designed and marketed the concept has lost its customer-friendly attitude. It may also hurt the company's reputation; as potential consumers might be unable to trust the company's judgement when it comes to AI models. In this way, evaluating the model is critical for avoiding the aforementioned side effects.

STEP 6: HYPERPARAMETER TUNING

On the off-chance that the evaluation is successful, we proceed to the hyperparameter tuning stage. This move aims to build on the encouraging results obtained during the assessment phase. For our model, we'd see if we could make it much superior at distinguishing between apples and mangos. There are many approaches we can take to improve the model. One of them is returning to the preparation step and preparing the model using different ranges of the preparation informational set. This can lead to greater precision, as the longer period of preparation allows for more openness and enhances the model's nature.

Another choice is to fine-tune the model's underlying qualities. As arbitrary starting values are perfected by experimentation, they often yield powerless outcomes. However, if we can come up with better introductory qualities or maybe start the model with a dissemination rather than a value, our outcomes may improve. We might play around with different boundaries to refine the model, but the interaction is more intuitive than sensible, so there is no clear technique for it.

STEP 7: PREDICTION

Expectation is the final step in the AI cycle. This is the point at which we assume the model is ready for practical use. Our natural product model should now be able to determine if a given natural product is an apple or a mango when asked. The model's final test would be whether it can outflank or, at the very least, organize human judgement in a variety of circumstances. The prediction step is what the end-client sees when they use the AI model within their specific industry. This evolution exemplifies why many people believe AI will be the ultimate fate of numerous companies.

7.4 TRAINING, TESTING AND VALIDATION

In projects that use supervised learning, a labelled dataset is built with labelled examples in which each and every observation consists of an output and one or more input variables. This dataset is divided into three parts, training set, testing set and validation set. This step is important for assessing the performance of the model and also to evaluate the effect of hyperparameter tuning. All these are the subsets of the original labelled dataset. The training set is used to train the model; this is fed into the algorithm, which then generates a model. The testing set is used to check the final performance of the model. It evaluates the performance by using some performance matrices and also gives an idea about the performance of different models (SVM, decision trees, KNN, neural network etc.) against each other. The third set of observations is called the validation or holdout set. This set is needed sometimes to tune the hyperparameters of the model with different values. Also, this set is used to detect overfitting. The division of the dataset is shown in Figure 7.2.

Some key points should be taken into consideration:

- In general, while splitting the dataset, 70%–90% of the data or the biggest part of the data is kept for training purposes and the remaining part of the dataset is divided into equal parts for testing and validation sets.

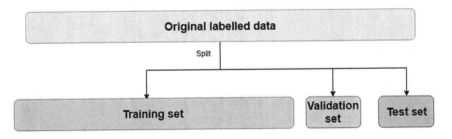

FIGURE 7.2 Division of labelled dataset.

- At the beginning of the project, test and validation sets are put aside and are not used for training.
- All three sets must contain diverse examples that address the problem. Also, there must be no overlapping between the data of the training and testing sets. This means one has to ensure that there is no observation which is common in both the datasets.

7.5   MACHINE LEARNING METHODS

Here, we discuss few major machine learning methods.

7.5.1   SUPERVISED LEARNING

A very popular approach used for the data classification and regression applications is "supervised learning." As the name suggests, the supervised model or machine is first trained by giving it examples and their interpretations. These interpretations may be categorical (for classification) or any real value (for regression problems). Once the model is trained, the unknown samples are given to it and, based on its previous knowledge, the model tries to map the inputs with the possible target values. Since the whole learning process of the machine is done in advance by examples and their respective outputs, this scheme is also known as "supervised machine learning." The major application area of supervised learning is in the field of medical data analysis where the machine learning model is trained by image or signal features, and later the model is able to detect or classify particular types of diseases like breast cancer, a brain tumour, epilepsy and so on. Some widely used supervised learning schemes are given in following sections.

NAIVE BAYES CLASSIFIER

The principle of the Bayesian classifier is to predict the value of a feature or features for all the members belonging to a certain class. So if a new object arrives with an unknown class, then the classifier can predict the object's class given some of its features. Classifier modelling is based on the probabilistic rule given by Bayes' theorem. The Bayes theorem of probability can be given as in Equation (7.1):

$$P(A/B) = \frac{P(B/A)P(A)}{P(B)},$$
(7.1)

where P(A/B) is the posterior probability, P(A) and P(B) are probabilities of the occurrence of event A and B respectively, and P(B/A) is the likelihood.

The naive Bayes classifier is a simple form of Bayesian classifier which assumes the impact of each feature independently for belonging in a particular class. The classifier assigns the membership of the test sample

$x \in X$ to the class y_i as [3]:

$$y_i = argmax \prod_{n=1}^{m} p\left(x_n | y_j\right), j = 1, 2, ...k,$$ (7.2)

where

m is the length of data points and
k is total class.

Although the naive Bayes classifier follows an independent assumption, it generally performs well even when the assumption is violated or not satisfied.

SUPPORT VECTOR MACHINE (SVM)

The SVM ML methods are popularly used techniques in addressing both classification as well as regression tasks. This is a kind of supervised method of ML in which classes of data samples are separated with the help of the construction of two hyperplanes implemented in parallel between the data points. The main aim of using this is to maximize the distance metric which is computed between the two hyperplanes, and the distance of either of the classes is maximized. The SVM is considered robust, easy to use and very well performing. The typical representation of SVM is shown in Figure 7.3.

The two hyperplanes that pass through one or more data points are known as boundary planes. The data points lying on these parallel boundary planes are called support vectors, and the distance between the boundary planes is called the margin. The best set of hyperplanes has the maximum margin between them. In the case of a non-linear classification problem, as shown in Figure 7.4, the linear classifier is unable to separate the candidates from the two classes properly. To handle this kind of situation, kernel functions are used which transform the input data space into some higher

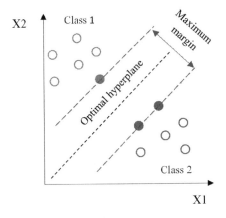

FIGURE 7.3   A support vector machine classifier.

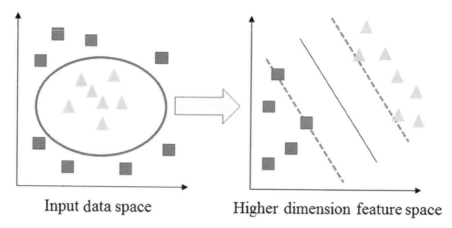

Input data space   Higher dimension feature space

FIGURE 7.4   Non-linear support vector machine.

dimension feature space where the points are linearly separable [4]. Commonly used kernel functions are: linear, radial basis function (RBF), and polynomial (of different orders). Mathematical details of SVM are given in the paragraphs below.

Let p be the number of data points, q be the number of features in data, y_i ($[y_{i1}, y_{i2} \ldots\ldots\ldots y_{iq}]$) be the vector which represents a data point in input space, z_i ($[z_{i1}, z_{i2}, \ldots\ldots\ldots z_{ip}]$) be the vector representing the target value of data points, and c ($[c_1, c_2, \ldots\ldots\ldots c_q]$) be the coefficient vector corresponding to the hyperplane. The objective of SVM is to find the hyperplane with the maximum margin, which takes the form:

$$c_1 y_1 + c_2 y_2 + \ldots\ldots\ldots + c_n y_n - d = 0, \tag{7.3}$$

where d is a scalar term generally known as bias.

The above equation can be rewritten as:

$$cy - d = 0. \tag{7.4}$$

The two parallel hyperplanes can be described by the following equations:

$$cy - d = 1 \text{ and} \tag{7.5}$$

$$cy - d = -1. \tag{7.6}$$

The distance between the hyperplanes separating the data points into two classes must be maximized to the possible extent. To exclude the data points, the bounding planes will now take the following form:

$$cy - d \geq 1 \text{ and} \tag{7.7}$$

$$cy - d \leq -1. \tag{7.8}$$

For a non-linear dataset, SVM transforms the data into higher dimensional space called feature space (ref. Figure 7.4), where a maximal separating hyperplane is constructed. Now, non-linear kernel functions are used to map the data into a feature space in a linear manner.

Some of the commonly used kernel functions are:

a. Linear kernel: $y_i^T \cdot y_j$

b. Polynomial kernel: $\left(y_i^T \cdot y_j + 1\right)^k$, where k is the degree of kernel.

c. Gaussian radial basis function (GRBF): $e^{-\gamma \|y_i - y_j\|_2}$, $\gamma = (2\sigma^2)^{-1}$, where σ is the parameter controlling the width of the kernel.

K-NEAREST NEIGHBOUR CLASSIFIER

K-nearest neighbour (K-NN) is a simple supervised classification scheme which looks for the similarity indexes with respect to the neighbours to classify a new test incident. Here, "K" is the number of neighbours of the test sample to be classified (a lower value of "K" increases the chances of a high classification error, whereas a higher value may require additional computational time). The neighbours are decided by a "distance metric" between the test sample and the components with already defined class labels. The components with shorter distances with the new element are considered as the neighbours. Generally, the number of neighbours is chosen to be odd (K = 3,5,7 etc.) to avoid conflicts between the two classes. Also, K-NN is a non-parametric algorithm, which means it does not make any assumption on the data that is being applied. Figure 7.5 shows how a new sample is classified according to a K-NN scheme. It can be clearly observed from the figure how the final response of the classifier changes when the value of "K" varies.

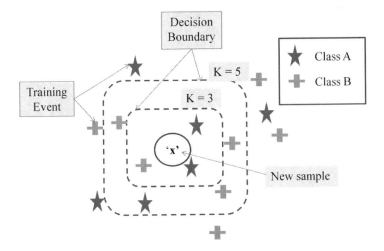

FIGURE 7.5 Schematic of K-NN classifier for K = 3 and K = 5.

There are different distance matrices utilized by the K-NN classifier in the process of finding the probable neighbours of the new event to be categorized. The most popular matrices are:

a) Euclidean Distance: The Euclidean distance metric is defined as follows:

$$d_E = \sqrt{\sum_{j=1}^{m} (x_j - y_j)^2},$$
(7.9)

where

m is the number of variables,
x and
y are the labelled and test incidents.

b) Manhattan Distance: The Manhattan distance metric is defined as follows:

$$d_M = \sum_{j=1}^{m} |x_j - y_j|.$$
(7.10)

c) Minkowski Distance: The Minkowski distance metric is defined as follows:

$$d_{Min} = \left(\sum_{j=1}^{m} \left(|x_j - y_j| \right)^q \right)^{1/q},$$
(7.11)

where q is generally calculated as sqrt (number of examples).

Example: The parameters of customers in a public bank database are given in the table below. Predict by using K-NN classifier whether a customer named "Manohar" belongs to the executive class or not.

Name	Loan Sanctioned	Income	No. of credit cards	Class
Rajiv	35L	35K	3	Yes
Balakrishna	22L	50K	2	No
Mukesh	63L	200K	1	Yes
Anil	59L	170K	1	Yes
Gautam	25L	40K	4	No
Manohar	37L	50K	2	No

Solution: Let us take Euclidean distance as the distance metric for this problem. Now, the distance between the parameters of "Manohar" and other customers will be calculated as follows:

- Distance between Rajiv and Manohar: sqrt[$(35 - 37)^2 + (35 - 50)^2 + (3 - 2)^2$] = 15.16.
- Distance between Balakrishna and Manohar: sqrt[$(22 - 37)^2 + (50 - 50)^2 + (2 - 2)^2$] = 15.
- Distance between Mukesh and Manohar: sqrt[$(63 - 37)^2 + (200 - 50)^2 + (1 - 2)^2$] = 152.23.
- Distance between Anil and Manohar: sqrt[$(59 - 37)^2 + (170 - 50)^2 + (1 - 2)^2$] = 122.
- Distance between Gautam and Manohar: sqrt[$(25 - 37)^2 + (40 - 50)^2 + (4 - 2)^2$] = 15.74.

The candidates with shorter distance matrices are "Rajiv," "Balakrishna" and "Gautam." Hence, they are considered as the neighbours of "Manohar." Now the class label of "Manohar" should belong to the class of these three candidates. The classes of "Rajiv," "Balakrishna" and "Gautam" are "Yes," "No" and "No." Since the majority class is "No," the k-NN classifier would therefore assign the class "No" to "Manohar."

DECISION TREE CLASSIFIER

The decision tree (DT) classifier is a simple, effective and widely used classification scheme. It applies a straightforward approach to solving any classification problem. The DT classifier defines a series of structured questions about the attributes of the test samples. Each time it arrives at a conditional response, and subsequently, a follow-up question is framed until a decision about the class label of the test event is made. There are a few popular algorithms which help create a DT based on the problem statements, for example, ID3, CART, and C4.5. The construction of DT may be based on binary or continuous numeric data with conditions, as shown in Figure 7.6 below.

In a DT, the initial root node with no incoming branch (in Figure 7.6(a), letter "C" and in Figure 7.6(b), "A < B") is considered a root node. All nodes except the root node (drawn with a circle in Figure 7.6(a) and (b)) are called internal nodes.

(a)

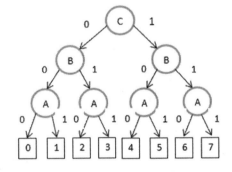

C	B	A	Output
0	0	0	0
0	0	1	1
0	1	0	2
0	1	1	3
1	0	0	4
1	0	1	5
1	1	0	6
1	1	1	7

FIGURE 7.6   Decision tree classifier (a) for binary data and (b) for numeric data.

(b)

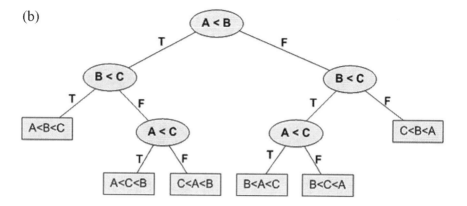

In rectangular boxes, we draw the nodes, and all such nodes are referred to as leaf or terminal nodes. The node edges, also called links, are resulted for a certain value of node. In a DT, the same value node is never repeated for a forward path. In addition, the DT does not have a unique structure due to the different ordering of internal nodes that produce a DT having different structures.

The ID3 algorithm is used in the DT, which means Iterative Dichotmiser 3. The ID3 is based on strategies of classification and a greedy approach is followed by the algorithm through selection of optimal parameters, which help in obtaining maximum information gain (IG) or minimum entropy (H). The steps involved in ID3 algorithms are:

1. Calculate entropy for dataset.
2. For each parameter: Calculate H for all its group values and IG for the feature.
3. Find the feature with maximum IG.
4. Repeat it until we get the tree.

A classification and regression tree (CART) is another popular approach to construct a classification as well as regression DT. CART is generally used to solve a multiple-class classification problem. It uses the Gini index (GI) as an evaluation metric for splitting a feature node in the DT. Steps of the CART algorithm are:

1. Select the root node based on the GI and maximum IG.
2. In each iteration, calculate the GI and IG considering that every node is used for the first time.
3. Split the whole dataset S to produce the subsets of data.
4. The algorithm follows recursion on each subset and on fresh attributes and creates the DT.

GI is mathematically defined as:

$$GI = 1 - \sum_{i=1}^{K} (p)^2, \tag{7.12}$$

where p is the probability of true condition and K is the total number of conditions.

The ID3 algorithm has certain shortcomings, such as there should be no missing value and the algorithm tends to overfit in some cases. An improved version of ID3 is the C4.5 algorithm, which overcomes the limitations of the ID3. During formation of the tree, the C4.5 selects the attribute which can split a set of samples in the most effective way in one class or the other. The splitting criterion used here is the normalized IG, and tree formation is started by the feature with the highest normalized IG. This process is then repeated further to make partitions and create sublists. The steps of C4.5 algorithms are:

1. For each attribute, C4.5 finds the normalized IG ratio by splitting between the features of the data.
2. Let X be that attribute with the highest normalized IG.
3. A decision node is created that splits on attribute X with others.
4. Recursion is performed in following steps, splitting the attributes and adds these nodes as children of the initial node.

RANDOM FOREST

The random forest (RF) is a classification algorithm which is constructed by incorporating many decision trees. For creating an uncorrelated bunch of trees, it uses bagging and feature randomness schemes while building an individual tree. The prediction of the committee of trees is considered to be more accurate than that of any individual tree. It suppresses the problem of overfitting that can occur in a single decision tree.

Bagging, or bootstrap aggregating, is a method of drawing a training set randomly for each decision tree from the training data. The size of each training set is equal to the original training size. This is done by a "features with replacement" strategy where some sample features are repeated and/or others are replaced. As the DT is very sensitive to the input training data, small changes in training sequence will offer a different and highly uncorrelated DT. In the end, the final outcome of the combination of DTs (random forest) is decided by majority vote. The RF classifier with bagging is shown in Figure 7.7.

Also, random selection pick from the overall set customizes the RF's tree in such a way that each tree will get different features to make the decision or create a "node." Hence, it increases between-the-trees variation significantly.

ARTIFICIAL NEURAL NETWORK (ANN)

An artificial neural network (ANN) is a technology-simulated model which follows the analogy of the human brain and the various function performed by the brain's neurons. One neuron communicates with the other by an entity known as a link. The neuron is sometimes known as a perceptron, and a neural network is also called as a multilevel perceptron model. The input is given to neurons or nodes which perform certain operations on that data.

The result of any node can be an output, or can be communicated to a different node. A general structure of a neural network with a single hidden layer is shown in

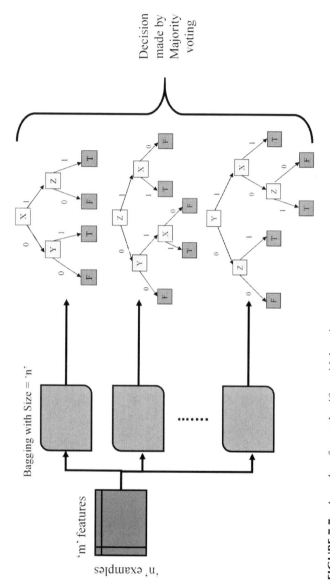

FIGURE 7.7　A random forest classifier with bagging.

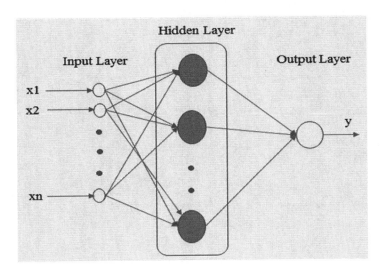

FIGURE 7.8   An artificial neural network model.

Figure 7.8 [4]. ANN follows the neuronal operation to process the given input. The output value of each node depends upon the weights of the links "w," inputs "x," bias "b" and node activation function " σ ." The equation of realization of a neural network can be given as:

$$z = wx^T + b. \qquad (7.13)$$

Here, "Z" is the logistic regression output. Next,

$$a = \sigma(z), \qquad (7.14)$$

where " a " is the output of activation function " σ " of the node which is applied on the output of Equation (7.13).

Therefore, it can be concluded from the above two equations that each node of the neural network performs two algebraic operations. Figure 7.9 displays the overall processing in the node.

Some examples of activation functions are:

1. Linear activation function

   The linear activation function is utilized to define the nature and interrelation of data. It is generally used in regression problems where the representation of data points is shown with the help of a line which covers (almost) all points. It can be represented by a straight line equation $y_1 = m_1 x$. The range of linear activation function is from $-\infty$ to $+\infty$.

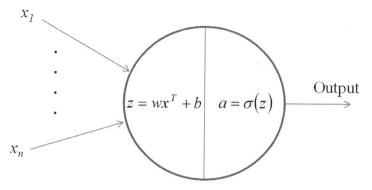

FIGURE 7.9   Node function of an artificial neural network.

2. Sigmoid function

This is an "S"-shaped activation function which ranges from 0 to 1. It is mainly used in the last layer of ANN in binary classification problems where the predicted class label is "0" or "1," or values between them. The equation of the sigmoid function is $y_1 = \dfrac{1}{\left(1+e^{-x}\right)}$.

3. Hyperbolic Tangent (Tanh)

The hyperbolic tangent function is the mathematically modified form of the sigmoid function. This function is usually used in the hidden layers of the complex neural networks.

   The range of values given by the "Tanh" function is between −1 and +1. Its mathematical form can be given as: $y_1 = \dfrac{2}{\left(1+e^{-2x}\right)} - 1$.

4. Relu activation function

Relu stands for "rectified linear unit." It is one of the most widely used functions for the picking of important features in the hidden layers of neural networks. This simple activation function can be defined as: $y_1 = max(0, x)$. The output of a "Relu" activation function is zero for all negative values of "x." Its output range is: [0, ∞).

   Example: Determine the class label of the input sample x = [−5 6] using a neural network. Given that bias = 1.2 and weights = [3 2], use the sigmoid activation function with the following conditions:

$$\text{Class} = \begin{cases} 0 \text{ if } a < 0.5; \\ 1 \text{ if } a \geq 0.5, \text{ where, "}a\text{" is the output of sigmoid activation function.} \end{cases}$$

Solution: Given parameters:

$$\text{Bias (b)} = 1.2$$

$$\text{Weights (w)} = [3 \; 2]$$

$$\text{Input (x)} = [-5 \; 6]$$

Therefore, from Equation (7.13),

$$z = \begin{bmatrix} 3 & 2 \end{bmatrix} \times \begin{bmatrix} -5 \\ 6 \end{bmatrix} + 1.2$$

$$= -1.8.$$

Now, from Equation (7.14), by applying the sigmoid activation function,

$$a = \frac{1}{1 + e^{-(-1.8)}}$$

$$= 0.14.$$

So, from the given conditions, the value of $a < 0.5$, the input sample therefore belongs to class-label = "0."

7.5.2 UNSUPERVISED LEARNING

It is not always necessary that the data comes with a label or class. In fact, most real-world datasets are depleted from their label. In that case, the machine is trained without any target value, merely on the basis of "data characteristics." The machine learns the inherent features possessed by the data and accordingly categorize it into two or more groups. It is important to take the note here that these machines do not define the class label of the data; rather, they simply separate the unlike samples from each other. Such kind of learning where the class or target value of the example is not predefined is known as "unsupervised learning." The models which perform the grouping or "clustering" task based on the interpretation of features or the nature of data without any external support or guidance are called unsupervised machine learning models. The descriptions of two popular algorithms of unsupervised category are:

K-MEANS CLUSTERING

Before diving directly into the concept of "k-means clustering," let us first understand what clustering is. Clustering is the grouping of data points from a large sample according to their similarities. For example, from a set of animals, two or more groups can be made on the basis of their attributes like weight, height, size and so on.

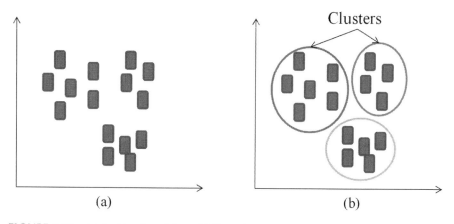

FIGURE 7.10   (a) Scatter plot of data. (b) Data clusters.

In general terms, clustering is done to understand and identify hidden patterns of the data. Figure 7.10 shows how the data points are grouped into clusters.

There are certain properties related to the cluster and its data points. First, all data points inside the cluster should share similar characteristics among them. For example, if it is a cluster of animals, then all "cats" should be grouped in the same cluster and so on. Second, samples belonging to different clusters show characteristics which should be as different as possible. For example, "cats" and "dogs" must be grouped in different clusters.

K-means clustering is a simple and very popular unsupervised learning scheme in which "k" is the number of clusters to be made in a given sample space. In Figure 7.10, the total three data clusters are there. In the k-means clustering method, the similarity index is measured in terms of "distance" of data points from the centre of the cluster. The cluster centre is also known as the "centroid." The value of "k" is generally assigned at the input side before processing of the data by the algorithm [5]. The k-means algorithm tries to minimize the sum of the distances between data points and the centroid of the cluster where they belong. The commonly used distance metric between the centroid and data points is defined as [5]:

$$d_{c,x} = \sqrt{\sum_{j=1}^{k}\sum_{i=1}^{n}\left(\mathbf{c}_j - \mathbf{x}_i\right)^2} \quad \forall\, n, \tag{7.15}$$

where "x" is the data vector, "n" is the number of data points, and "c" is the centroid of a cluster.

The steps involved in the processing of the k-means clustering method are given in the below points.

1. Initialize the number of cluster "k."
2. Select "k" cluster centroids randomly among data points.

3. Calculate the distances of all data points with the cluster centres and assign the points to the respective cluster for which the distance became minimum.
4. After no points are left to assign, recompute the new clusters' centroids.
5. Repeat steps 3 and 4 until the stopping criteria are met.

There are mainly three criteria which can be utilized to stop further progressing of the k-means algorithm:

a. If the new cluster centres are same as the previous ones.
b. If the data points of the clusters remain the same.
c. When the maximum number of iterations is reached.

Example: With the help of the k-means clustering algorithm, arrange the customers given in the below table of a private sector bank into two different groups. Follow the standard stopping criteria of the k-means algorithm.

Customer	Income (in lac.)	Debt (in lac.)
C1	1	1
C2	2	1
C3	4	3
C4	5	4

Solution: Given that: k = 2 and number of attributes = 2 (Income, Debt)
    Now, to visualize the above data, we first represent it in terms of a scatter plot as follows:

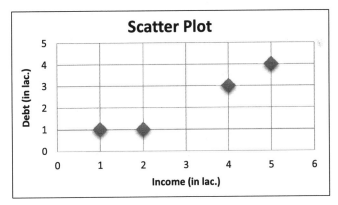

Let us assume that the initial cluster centres (centroids) are: c1(1,1) and c2(2,1).
    Now, calculate the distance from centroid c1 to each data point with the help of Equation (15):

$$d1: \sqrt{(1-1)^2 + (1-1)^2} = 0, \quad d2: \sqrt{(1-2)^2 + (1-1)^2} = 1,$$

$$d3: \sqrt{(1-4)^2 + (1-3)^2} = 3.61, \text{ and } d4: \sqrt{(1-5)^2 + (1-4)^2} = 5.$$

Similarly, for centroid c2,

$$\text{d1: } \sqrt{(2-1)^2 + (1-1)^2} = 1, \text{ d2: } \sqrt{(2-2)^2 + (1-1)^2} = 0,$$

$$\text{d3: } \sqrt{(2-4)^2 + (1-3)^2} = 2.83, \text{ and d4: } \sqrt{(2-5)^2 + (1-4)^2} = 4.24.$$

So, in combined form:

$$d = \begin{bmatrix} 0 & 1 & 3.61 & 5 \\ 1 & 0 & 2.83 & 4.24 \end{bmatrix} \begin{bmatrix} c1(group1) \\ c2(group2) \end{bmatrix}$$

Now, from the minimum distance policy, it is clear from the above distance matrix that only point (1,1) belongs to c1; the rest of the points belong to c2.

The next step is to determine the new centroids:

Since group 1 has only one member, the centroid remains the same for it, that is, c1 = (1,1).

For group 2, the new centroid is calculated as $c2 = \left(\dfrac{2+4+5}{3}, \dfrac{1+3+4}{3} \right) = (3.67, 2.67)$.

Again, the distance matrix for the new centroids by following a similar approach for all points would be:

$$d = \begin{bmatrix} 0 & 1 & 3.61 & 5 \\ 3.14 & 2.36 & 0.47 & 1.89 \end{bmatrix} \begin{bmatrix} c1(group1) \\ c2(group2) \end{bmatrix}$$

So, from the minimum distance policy, now points (1,1) and (2,1) belong to group 1 and points (4,3) and (5,4) belong to group 2.

New centroids for the next step will be:

$$c1 = \left(\frac{1+2}{2}, \frac{1+1}{2} \right) = (1.5, 1) \text{ and } c2 = \left(\frac{4+5}{2}, \frac{3+4}{2} \right) = (4.5, 3.5).$$

For these new centroids, the distance matrix would be:

$$d = \begin{bmatrix} 0.5 & 0.5 & 3.2 & 4.61 \\ 4.3 & 3.54 & 0.71 & 0.71 \end{bmatrix} \begin{bmatrix} c1(group1) \\ c2(group2) \end{bmatrix}$$

Therefore, from the minimum distance policy, again points (1,1) and (2,1) belong to group 1, and points (4,3) and (5,4) belong to group 2.

Since there is no alteration in group members and therefore the k-means algorithm converges here. Hence, the group or cluster distribution of the customers would be as follows:

Customer	Income (in lac.)	Debt (in lac.)	Group
C1	1	1	1
C2	2	1	1
C3	4	3	2
C4	5	4	2

FUZZY C-MEANS CLUSTERING

The fuzzy c-means (FCM) clustering approach is similar to k-means clustering except that here, each and every data point is associated with all available clusters instead of a single one. The association of a data point with all the clusters is defined by likelihoods corresponding to all clusters, which show how much the data point does belong to each and every cluster. FCM is a very popular clustering method for solving problems, especially in the field of medical science where it is necessary to group unlabelled data based on their internal characteristics. This technique is based on expectation-minimization of the least-squared function as given by [6]:

$$J_m = \sum_{j=1}^{k} \sum_{i=1}^{n} \mu_{ij}^m \left\| c_j - x_i \right\|^2,$$

where "m" is the real exponent with any value greater than 1. μ_{ij} is the membership weight of point x_i belongs to cluster c_j.

The steps involved in the FCM algorithm are given below [6]:

1. Initialize the membership matrix $\mu = \mu_{ij}$ as μ^0

2. Calculate the centroid as $c_j = \dfrac{\sum\limits_{i=1}^{n} \mu_{ij}^m \times x_i}{\sum\limits_{i=1}^{n} \mu_{ij}^m}$.

3. Update the membership matrix by the following equation:

$$\mu_{ij}^+ = \frac{1}{\sum\limits_{k=1}^{c} \left(\dfrac{\left\| c_j - x_i \right\|}{\left\| c_k - x_i \right\|} \right)^{\frac{2}{m-1}}} .$$

4. If the change in updated and previous values is small enough, that is, $\left\| \mu^+ - \mu \right\| \leq \delta$, then the algorithm converges.

7.6   PERFORMANCE EVALUATION OF MACHINE LEARNING MODEL

We can assess the performance of our designed model based on a number of parameters. Let's take a quick look at each of them.

Confusion Matrix: This is essentially an NXN matrix that stores information about the real and expected values of data inputs, with N denoting the number of target classes. It's the simplest and most effective way to represent and analyse a classification-based model.

The confusion matrix includes four important parameters, whose brief descriptions are as follows:

- **True Positives (TP)** – This is the case when the predicted cases become the actual cases and thus the prediction of cases being true is correct. The condition "true," or positive, is also denoted by 1.
- **True Negatives (TN)** – In this case, the predicted values claimed as true actually become false and thus a true negative is the outcome. So, the actual as well as predicted values become 0.
- **False Positives (FP)** – If the predicted value is 1 and the actual value becomes 0, then the prediction is false. Such a case is called a false positive.
- **False Negatives (FN)** – In this case, the predicted value is 0 and the actual value is 1, and thus a false negative results.

A confusion matrix plays an important role especially in the computation of classification performance using a ML technique. This is also referred to as sklearn.metric for the evaluation of the performance of various classification models

Accuracy: For classification algorithms, accuracy is the most used performance metric. It's the number of accurate forecasts divided by the total number of predictions. With the help of the following formula, we can easily compute it using a confusion matrix:

$$Accuracy = (TP + TN) / (TP + FP + FN + TN)... \qquad (7.16)$$

To calculate the accuracy of our classification model, we can use the accuracy score function in sklearn.metric.

Classification Report: Precisions, Recall, F1, and Support scores are included in this report. The following are the explanations:

Precision: The number of correct documents returned by our ML model can be specified as precision in document retrievals.

$$Precision = TP / (TP + FP)... \qquad (7.17)$$

Recall or Sensitivity: The number of positives returned by our ML model is known as recall. With the help of the following formula, we can easily compute it using the confusion matrix.

$$Recall = TP / (TP + FN)... \qquad (7.18)$$

Specificity: In contrast to recall, specificity can be defined as the number of negatives returned by our machine learning model.

$$Specificity = TN / (TN + FP)... \qquad (7.19)$$

Support: The support is defined as the possibility of falling the response into each class of target where the true response in contributed by the number of samples.

F1 Score: The F1 score is the weighted average of accuracy and recall in mathematics. We get the harmonic mean of accuracy and recall from this score. F1 has a best value of 1 and a worst value of 0. The following formula can be used to compute the F1 score:

$$F1 = 2 * \frac{(precision * recall)}{(precision + recall)}... \qquad (7.20)$$

Precision and recall both contribute equally to the F1 score. To get the classification report of our classification model, we can use the classification report function of sklearn.metrics.

AUC (Area Under ROC curve): This is also known as the AUC-ROC curve, which indicates the performance of classification that is done on different values of threshold. The ROC here is the receiver operating characteristic, and a probability curve. The AUC measures the separability, which means that various classes are differentiated and the ability to distinguish is indicated by the AUC-ROC curve. The greater the value of the AUC, the better the model used, whose value can be calculated from the plot highlighting the relationship between true positive rate (TPR) and false positive rate (FPR), in other words, the specificity values at different values of threshold. The ROC score function is used for calculating AUC-ROC, from sklearn metrics.

	Actual Values	
	Positive (1)	**Negative (0)**
Positive (1)	TP	FP
Negative (0)	FN	TN

Predicted Values

FIGURE 7.11   Confusion matrix representation.

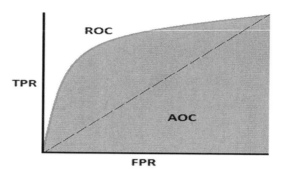

FIGURE 7.12 Representation of ROC-AUC curve.

Figure 7.12 shows a typical ROC-AUC curve which depicts a graph having ROC and AUC as values.

LEARNING OUTCOMES

After studying this chapter, the students will be able to:

- Explain the importance of machine learning in medical image diagnosis and applications
- Enumerate a few important methods of ML
- Explain ML-based classifiers
- Distinguish between supervised and unsupervised ML techniques

EXERCISE

Q1. What do we mean by the terms underfitting and overfitting?

Q2. Explain the different steps of machine learning.

Q3. How can we assess the performance of a machine learning model?

Q4. What do we mean by confusion matrix?

Q5. How do we choose a suitable machine learning method? Discuss the performance metrics involved in evaluating the classifiers.

REFERENCES

1. Samuel, A. L. (1959). Some studies in machine learning. *IBM Journal of Research and Development, 3*(3), 210–229.
2. Mitchell, T. M. (1997). *Machine learning.* McGraw Hill.
3. Theodoridis, S., & Koutroumbas, K. (2009). *Pattern recognition.* 2009.
4. Atrey, K., Sharma, Y., Bodhey, N. K., & Singh, B. K. (2019). Breast cancer prediction using dominance-based feature filtering approach: A comparative investigation in machine learning archetype. *Brazilian Archives of Biology and Technology, 62.* https://doi.org/10.1590/1678-4324-2019180486

5. Übeyli, E. D., & Doğdu, E. (2012). Erratum to: Automatic detection of erythemato-squamous diseases using k-means clustering. *Journal of Medical Systems, 36*(2), 1007. https://doi.org/10.1007/s10916-010-9534-8

6. Singh, B. K., Verma, K., & Thoke, A. S. (2016). Fuzzy cluster based neural network classifier for classifying breast tumors in ultrasound images. *Expert Systems with Applications, 66*, 114–123.

8 Cancer Detection
Breast Cancer Detection Using Mammography, Ultrasound and Magnetic Resonance Imaging (MRI)

LEARNING OBJECTIVES

The chapter aims to cover:

- Need for breast cancer screening and diagnosis
- Modalities used in breast cancer treatment
- Comparison of modalities
- Role of machine learning in computer-aided diagnosis (CAD)
- Performance evaluation of CAD system

Breast cancer is among the second major cause of death in women worldwide. To decrease the mortality rates, early diagnosis plays an important role in medical imaging. Breast cancer is detected with the help of mammogram and ultrasound, and lesions or micro-calcifications are segmented. The segmented results are classified into cancerous and non-cancerous regions. The use of soft computing methods has made cancer detection easier, more efficient and optimal. Machine learning (ML) techniques are very effective ways to classify data and thus used in diagnosis and decision-making. In this chapter, various screening techniques employed to detect breast cancer are discussed. Also, we present a review of work done by various research contributions that implemented machine learning approaches in breast cancer diagnosis.

8.1 INTRODUCTION

Breast cancer (BC) is amongst the most commonly diagnosed cancers in women worldwide. It is the second leading cause of cancer-related deaths in women world-wide, and study suggests that the mortality rate is highest due to breast cancer deaths in women, especially those in the age group 20–59 [1]. In 2019, an estimated 268,600 new cases of invasive breast cancer were diagnosed among women in the United States [2]. Moreover, 276,480 new cases are estimated for the year 2020 [3]. Breast cancer usually starts in the inner lining of the milk ducts or the lobules that supply them with milk. Broadly, the tumours are classified as two types, benign (non-cancerous) and malignant (cancerous). Different screening methods available for the

DOI: 10.1201/9781003097808-8

diagnosis of breast cancer include mammography, ultrasound (US), and magnetic resonance imaging (MRI). X-ray mammography is considered the most effective technique for early detection of breast cancer and routine breast cancer screening. For dense breasts as well as in women having surgical interventions, the reliability of cancer detection is a major concern. Several studies have proved that US and MRI are better alternatives to mammography in certain cases, and because this modality does involve radiation exposure [4].

8.2   DIFFERENT IMAGING MODALITIES

Medical image processing is a specific area of image processing and has a number of modalities, which means there are various types of medical images. The modalities used for breast cancer detection are briefly discussed here.

8.2.1   MAMMOGRAPHY (MG)

In the mammography method, we use X-rays for generating breast images as mammograms [5]. Early detection using screening with mammography can help reduce the mortality rate among women. The procedure is applied and screening is done in different views, two for each breast, namely, the craniocaudal (CC) view and the mediolateral oblique (MLO) view [5]. The MLO projection is carried out by placing the object generally at an angle of 45° or any other value in between 30° and 60°. The CC projection is obtained using a vertical X-ray beam [1]. The MLO and CC views are shown in Figure 8.1 for the left breast highlighting a malignant tumour [6, 7]. Among mammography techniques, modern screening and clinical procedure mainly involves digital mammography (DM), which helps in segmentation of the classification of cancerous elements in breast tissues. Tumours are detected before

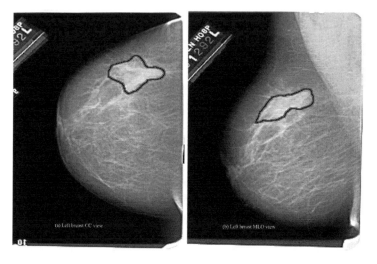

FIGURE 8.1   Different views used in mammography [6, 7].

the symptoms actually appear and are seen by the radiologists and physicians. The smallest variations in micro-calcification or calcium deposits are detected by the DM technique for early diagnosis of breast cancer [8].

Several research papers and articles are reported in the literature for the detection of masses and micro-calcifications used in various types of breast cancer segmentation and classification. Dheeba et al. (2014) [9] investigated a classification approach for the detection of abnormalities in digital mammograms of breast images with the help of the particle swarm optimized wavelet neural network (PSOWNN). The texture energy measures were extracted from the images and applied the resulting patterns to the classifier for classifying the suspicious regions. With the proposed approach, a ROC of 0.96853 was obtained. Singh and Urooj (2016) [10] presented a computer-aided-diagnosis (CAD) system to classify breast tissues. For the texture descriptors, pseudo-Zernike moments (GPZM) and pseudo-Zernike moments (PZM) were utilized. For improving classification accuracy, an adaptive differential evolution wavelet neural network (Ada-DEWNN) was implemented as a classifier.

Hariraj et al. (2018) [11] evaluated the performance of the Fuzzy-Multi layer SVM (FMSVM) classifier on mammographic images of the breast. This method resulted in an accuracy of 98% for the detection of malignant, benign and normal tumours. Sokary et al. (2019) [12] suggested CAD-based breast cancer detection which employs mammograms and uses the Gaussian mixture model (GMM) for enhancement of the mammograms; and the results of GMM are further subjected to a support vector machine (SVM) for classification. A classification accuracy of 92.5% is achieved and benign and malignant tissues are separated. Alqudah et al. (2019) [13] developed a CAD system to perform automatic segmentation. The classification of breast masses into seven classes is performed using a probabilistic neural network (PNN) with an accuracy of 97.08%. Another classification into the benign and malignant category is done using support vector machine (SVM) with an accuracy of 99.18%. Singh et al. (2019) [14] performed segmentation using various techniques, such as expected maximization, K-means, Fuzzy c-Means (FCM), multilevel thresholding, region growing (RG), and particle swarm optimization (PSO). Vanderheyden et al. (2020) [15] developed a classifier based on a deep learning method called Ordinal Hyperplane Loss-all centroids (OHPLall) that predicts malignancy rates as per the Breast Imaging Reporting and Data System (BI-RADS) category. This shows that it can help radiologists as a supplementary tool in breast cancer diagnosis.

8.2.2 ULTRASOUND (US)

Ultrasound is one of the modalities used by radiologists and physicians for examination of the breast to detect and diagnose the possible presence of cancerous masses. The ultrasound modality of the breast is considered an indispensable tool in breast imaging methods [1]. This method of imaging produces the proper output for women who have dense breasts, which helps in the efficient detection of masses. This is a non-invasive method of breast imaging, referred to as breast ultrasound, and used for detection of micro-calcifications or masses [16] in all cases of suspected breast images. Ultrasound is highly sensitive in differentiating benign breast lesions from malignant ones [5]. Ultrasound helps calculate the tumour size and characterize abnormalities

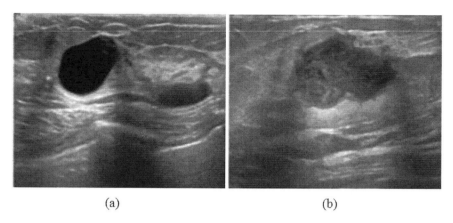

(a)   (b)

FIGURE 8.2 Breast ultrasound images showing (a) Benign tumour (b) Malignant tumour [17].

detected by digital mammography (DM) [8]. Breast masses are classified as malignant or benign depending on the structure, shape, texture and other geometric properties. High-frequency sound signals are used for the production of breast ultrasound images that highlight the tissues of the breast, unlike X-ray images, where X-rays are used for imaging. Breast ultrasound is considered a good modality because it is cost effective and easily accessible. Breast ultrasound is preferred over mammography due its capability of detecting cancerous areas that were not seen in mammograms or when performing a physical examination [5]. The lesions inside breast images can be distinguished explicitly in breast ultrasound images and benign elements can be separated from malignant masses. Malignant masses cannot be ignored which can cause cancer, whereas benign ones can be ignored. The difference between different masses inside the breast is measured in terms of some appropriate features, which may be of statistical and dimensional types. Generally, non-uniformity is dominantly present in the case of benign masses, and the description of masses is made using lobulations, margins, different axes and so on. There are different features for identifying malignancy in breast images and their descriptions are made by speculated margins, microlobulated margins, acoustic shadowing, micro-calcifications and so on. Cancerous masses are hypoechoic in response to bright echogenic fibroglanular tissue. Breast ultrasound images having benign and malignant masses or lesions can be seen in Figure 8.2 [17].

Sonography is regarded as an important imaging modality for the diagnosis of breast lesions. Abdelwahed et al. (2015) [18] proposed a computer-aided diagnosis (CAD) system for the segmentation and classification of breast cancer in ultrasound images. Various classifiers like SVM, K-nearest neighbour (KNN), and classification and regression trees (CART) were used. A classification accuracy of 100% was obtained using texture features that were subjected to SVM and CART classifiers.

Flores et al. (2015) [19] suggested a classification approach that combines texture and morphological features, and feature selection is appropriately made based on statistical features and mutual information. The local fisher discriminant analysis (LFDA) method is used for classification and an AUC (area under ROC curve where ROC is the region of convergence) of 0.942 is obtained for a linear kernel utilizing five feature sets of morphological features. A CAD technique for segmentation and classification of mass in ultrasound images was proposed by Menon et al. (2015) [20]. The dimensionality of features was reduced using principal component analysis (PCA), and an accuracy of 95.7% for classification was obtained using SVM as classifier. Xian et al. (2015) [21] implemented the segmentation of breast ultrasound (BUS) images, an accurate region of interest (ROI) was extracted, and tumour areas were segmented from BUS images effectively. The segmentation method utilizes edge-related information in the frequency domain in addition to other intensity-related information such as an intensity distribution profile, position, pose and so on in the spatial domain. The performance of the model is evaluated using the area and boundary error metrics. Gu et al. (2016) [22] proposed an automated algorithm to segment 3D ultrasound images into three major types of tissue. Using the overlap ratio, an average similarity of 74.54 % was obtained. Shan et al. (2016) [23] proposed the use of Breast Imaging Reporting and Data System (BI-RADS) features and machine learning techniques (like SVM, random forest) for the computer-aided diagnosis of breast ultrasound images. Singh et al. (2016, 2017) [24, 25] performed classification on breast ultrasound images using SVM and a back-propagation artificial neural network (BPANN) as classifiers to categorize breast tumours as benign or malignant.

Luo et al. (2017) [26] presented a breast image segmentation method that combines edge- and region-based information, and the performance of segmentation was made optimal with the help of the particle swarm optimization (PSO) method. The segmentation is referred to as the robust graph-based (RGB) segmentation method. Liu et al. (2018) [27] proposed a computational framework that can detect and segment breast lesions in a fully automatic manner and which can operate to whole ultrasound images. The Otsu-based adaptive thresholding (OBAT) algorithm was implemented to locate tumour regions and initialize tumour contours, and finally, the Chan-Vese model method was used. Uzunhisarcikli and Goreke (2018) [28] developed a classifier model based on Type-2 fuzzy inference to classify a breast tumour as benign or malignant using the BI-RADS category. Daoud et al. (2019) [29] suggested an automatic BUS segmentation which operates on sub-pixels that are obtained by decomposition of the entire image, maintaining edge-related information and high boundary recall ratio. The performance was evaluated in terms of the detection rate, which is computed by using true positive (TP), false positive (FP), false negative (FN), and similarity ratios.

Panigrahi et al. (2019) [30] developed a clustering-based segmentation technique called the multi-scale Gaussian kernel induced fuzzy C-means (MsGKFCM) method for breast ultrasound images. Kozegar et al. (2019) [31] carried out a survey on computer-aided detection (CADe) in 3D breast ultrasound images. Virmani and Agarwal (2019) [32] designed a CAD system for classification of breast tumours by considering the effect of de-speckle filtering in breast ultrasound images. Lyu and Wang (2019) [33] suggested the use of ultrasound imaging as a necessary supplement to X-ray imaging of the breast for distinguishing cysts from solid tumours and examining dense breasts. An anisotropic diffusion algorithm (MAD) is suggested based on the most frequent filtering (MFF). Xu et al. (2019) [34] proposed the use of convolutional neural networks (CNNs) for the segmentation of breast ultrasound images. In a study proposed by Chang et al. (2020) [35], several features related to the BI-RADS category were selected and machine learning classifiers like SVM, random forest (RF), and convolution neural network (CNN) were used to perform classification.

8.2.3 Magnetic Resonance Imaging (MRI)

MRI is used in the diagnosis of breast, brain and other abnormalities of human body. The MRI has as its variant f-MRI (functional MRI), which is a very important modality for the analysis of brain disorders and functionalities. In breast cancer detection, MRI is considered a fast-emerging area of medical imaging which helps in good visibility of lesions and masses in the breast. In MRI, during the screening process, the image is converted into a number of slices and thus the detection of masses becomes easier. The entire volume of the breast structure is covered by the image modality. High-risk women are generally recommended to undergo MRI screening, which simplifies the assessment of therapy and post-detection of masses [8]. The suspected areas are emphasized by MRI, and therefore this modality supplements BUS and mammograms if any difficulty is reported in these modalities. The sensitivity of the imaging method is very high, in the range 89–100% for invasive cases, but the value of specificity is not high (generally, up to 72%). The sensitivity and specificity are used as criteria for performance assessment of the CAD system, which is used to highlight malignant lesions [5]. The MRI carries a lot of information with it which needs proper interpretation, and this is done by using machine learning techniques. The breast regions can be very accurately classified and segregated with the help of machine learning methods.

Kuhl et al. (2017) [36] investigated the use and accuracy of breast magnetic resonance (MR) imaging as a supplemental screening tool to investigate the cancer type detected using MRI screening. For women at average risk of breast cancer, MRI screening improves early diagnosis of breast cancer. Dalmis et al. (2018) [37] implemented deep learning to develop a computer-aided detection (CADe) system which uses the spatial information obtained from MRI scans. The proposed system obtained an average sensitivity of 0.6429 ± 0.0537. Venkata et al. (2019) [38] studied the effectiveness of the imaging modalities and systems used for breast cancer diagnosis. The study involved all modalities BUS, mammograms and MRI, and logical regression was used as a machine learning method in the diagnosis process for breast cancer. MRI was found to exhibit better sensitivity performance in comparison with two other modalities, ultrasound and mammograms. Herent et al. (2019) [39] developed a lesion-characterization model for MR images. They obtained a weighted mean area under the curve (AUC) of 0.816 for test data. The major limitations of breast MRI include low specificity and also its interpretation is complex; hence, it is recommended mostly for the screening of high-risk women. Further, it is costly, time-consuming, and it cannot be performed on patients with pacemakers, cochlear implants, iron-based metal implants and so on [4].

TABLE 8.1
Assessment Categories of BI-RADS

Category	Assessment	Finding	Follow-up Recommendation
0	Incomplete	Need additional imaging evaluation and/or prior mammograms for comparison	Additional imaging and/or obtain prior images for comparison
1	Complete	Negative	Routine screening mammograms
2		Benign finding(s)	Routine screening mammograms
3		Probably benign finding	Follow-up 6-month mammogram
4		Suspicious abnormality Optional subdivisions: 4A: Low suspicion for malignancy 4B: Intermediate suspicion of malignancy 4C: Moderate concern, but not classic for malignancy	Biopsy should be considered
5	Complete	Highly suggestive of malignancy	Biopsy required
6		Known biopsy-proven malignancy	Appropriate action should be taken

8.3 BREAST IMAGING REPORTING AND DATA SYSTEM (BI-RADS)

A standard system of imaging, reporting and data analysis is the Breast Imaging Reporting and Data System (BI-RADS®) owned by the American College of Radiology (ACR) that helps in the reporting of breast pathology of mammography, ultrasound and magnetic resonance imaging (MRI). Its initial edition was created in 1993 and the fifth edition of BI-RADS was released in 2013 [40]. The various categories of classification and assessment of reporting can be effectively made by this system. These assessment categories and recommendations are presented in Table 8.1.

8.4 USEFULNESS OF MACHINE LEARNING (ML)

As we know, machine learning has become an essential part of all automated analysis and diagnosis systems of medical imaging, and this is the case in cancer detection as well. ML techniques are used for extracting a suitable number of features by training the data, and the features are further used for classification and segmentation of different regions of the breast or any other medical images while diagnosing the presence of cancer. Supervised and unsupervised categories of ML techniques are mainly studied in various literatures [41]. In unsupervised learning, no prior

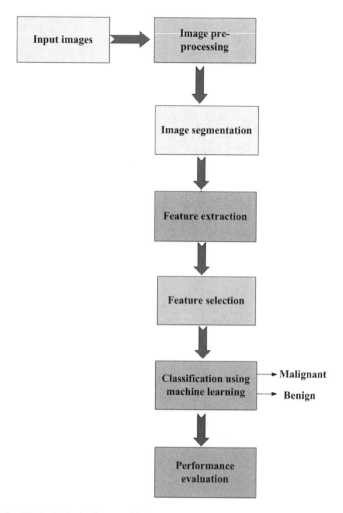

FIGURE 8.3   Typical block diagram highlighting steps for breast cancer detection.

information is given to the training process and feature extraction, and classification is made, whereas in supervised learning methods of ML, the parameters of algorithms or methods are adjusted in such a manner so that an optimal or known output results. In Figure 8.3, different steps in breast cancer detection can be seen and all major stages of the block diagram shown in Figure 8.3 are discussed here briefly.

8.4.1   IMAGE PRE-PROCESSING

This step is very important and used to remove unwanted noise and other artefacts from the image acquired using various imaging systems before applying any further processing. In a few reported studies, the CAD system was designed for classification, and de-speckle filtering was studied by Virmani and Agarwal (2019) [32].

Also, an anisotropic diffusion algorithm (MAD) was implemented by Lyu and Wang (2019) [33] on breast ultrasound images. Some other pre-processing techniques such as histogram equalization, anisotropic diffusion, linear filtering and Wiener filtering are commonly applied for the enhancement of the images.

8.4.2 IMAGE SEGMENTATION

This step is considered a vital step in the development of an efficient CAD system. The separation of the region of interest (ROI) is the main purpose of segmentation. The segmentation technique extracts the tumour from an image which is used for further examination. Segmentation is a process of partitioning an image into its specific parts and extracting the region of interest to perform further analysis. Image segmentation finds promising applications in the field of medical imaging, and used in analysis of anatomical tissues for later quantitative analysis. Usually, image segmentation is carried out by taking into consideration the colour information of the image, greyscale, edge, texture and other spatial information.

The processing of images manually is a laborious task and requires much time without the use of powerful optimization techniques. A few authors have proposed methods for segmentation combining both region- and edge-based information. Luo et al. (2017) [26] used an RGB segmentation method, and automatic segmentation was implemented by Daoud et al. (2019) [29] on breast ultrasound images. Singh et al. (2019) [14] implemented expected maximization, K-means, FCM, multilevel thresholding, RG and PSO. Active contours, watershed segmentation, graph cuts and clustering are some other common techniques applied [42] for segmentation, as shown in Figure 8.4.

8.4.3 FEATURE EXTRACTION

In the feature extraction step, several features related to the characteristics of the lesions are extracted from the medical image. The features are used to distinguish between benign and malignant tumours. Image features mainly refer to the attributes or properties of an image such as edges, texture, colour and so on. Commonly used features of an image include shape, texture and colour. When compared to other features, the colour feature is invariant to rotation angle and scale, is generally fast, and offers stronger stability. Texture features are used to describe the surface properties of an image. The most commonly used texture features are employed to describe the texture features that include the grey-level co-occurrence matrix, wavelet transform, Gabor filter representation and so on. The shape features such as area, perimeter and so on are used to describe the shape characteristics (edges and regions) of the objects in an image. From mammograms of breast images, texture energy measures are easily extracted in Dheeba et al. (2014) [9]. In Singh et al. (2016) [10], pseudo-Zernike moments (PZM) are used as texture descriptors. Figure 8.5 shows the various types of features extracted from ROI which play a vital role in classification. We can see that features are mainly three types, shape, texture and colour based.

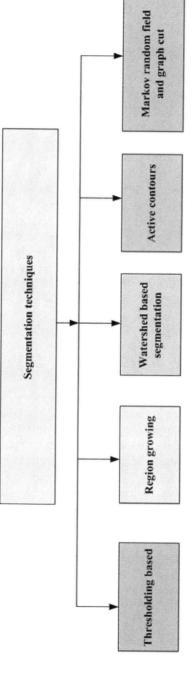

FIGURE 8.4   Different types of image segmentation techniques.

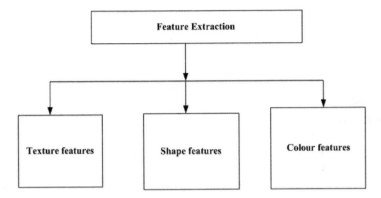

FIGURE 8.5 Commonly extracted type of features.

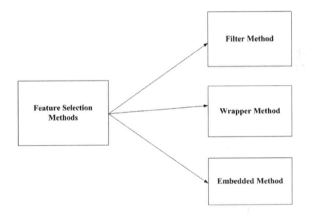

FIGURE 8.6 Types of feature selection techniques.

8.4.4 FEATURE SELECTION

Usually, a very large feature set may lead to more computational time, and also the accuracy of classification may get affected due to redundant features. Hence, feature selection [31, 35] is a step carried out to select the most effective features. A large number of features in the dataset increases the risk of overfitting in the model. Hence, several feature selection techniques are employed to reduce these feature dimensions without much loss in the information. Various types of feature selection techniques are available like filter method, wrapper method and embedded method. Figure 8.6 shows the various techniques implemented for the selection of relevant features. In the filter method, the performance of each feature is evaluated by correlating it with the target, whereas in the wrapper-based approach, the best combination of variables is obtained using various methods like subset selection, forward stepwise selection and backward stepwise selection. In the embedded method, less important predictors are assigned low weight.

8.4.5 CLASSIFICATION

The classification of the suspicious lesion into a benign or malignant category is performed using machine learning techniques. Classification plays an important role in the diagnosis of breast cancer. Hence, the selection of a reliable classifier is critical for distinguishing benign breast tumours from malignant ones [42]. The purpose of designing a classifier using machine learning is to train a classification model to automatically perform classification into different classes, thereby minimizing the error for all training samples. Various types of classifiers are used by different researchers to perform the classification task. In machine learning, basically two types of techniques, supervised and unsupervised learning, are implemented, as shown in Figure 8.7. In supervised learning, the model is trained with known input

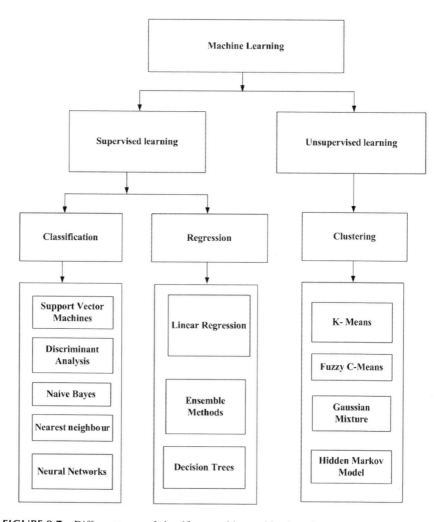

FIGURE 8.7 Different types of classifiers used in machine learning.

and output data to predict future outputs. In the supervised learning method or algorithm, we use known input data, and the output data or response is also known; and to get the desired output, the training continues. The training generates a number of predicted data, but the output which is nearest the desired data output is chosen. The predictive models under the supervised method of learning are mainly classification and regression methods. Classification models classify input data like whether a tumour is malignant or benign. Regression techniques predict continuous responses. In the unsupervised learning method, input data is known but no any labelled data output or response is provided, and thus the training process gets inferences from the input data itself. A number of hidden patterns are generated in this method. Clustering is the most popular and commonly used example under this type of ML.

Sokary et al. (2019) [12] proposed machine learning-based classifiers like SVM, and BPANN was implemented by Singh et al. (2017) [25]. Random forest was implemented by Shan et al. (2016) [23], while Abdelwahed et al. (2015) [18] used KNN and classification and regression trees to perform classification of breast ultrasound and mammography images. Also, logistic regression was used by Venkata and Lingamgunta (2019) [38] to evaluate imaging techniques (US, MG, MRI) to diagnose breast cancer. Several types of classifiers are used in machine learning to perform the classification of breast lesions. Figure 8.7 shows the most commonly used classifiers.

8.4.6   PERFORMANCE EVALUATION

The confusion matrix gives the values of true positive (TP), false positive (FP), true negative (TN), and false negative (FN). The various performance metrics like classification accuracy, sensitivity, specificity, the area under the curve (AUC), and so on can be computed to evaluate the performance of the classifier.

Figure 8.8 shows the detailed block diagram approach used for the implementation of machine learning for the diagnosis of breast cancer. Images of different modalities like mammography, ultrasonography and MRI are used. To reduce the effect of noise and other artefacts, pre-processing of acquired images can be done. This will help correct background illumination as well. After pre-processing, the selection of the region of interest, that is, locating the tumour and /or lesion, will be carried out to perform segmentation. Feature extraction is carried out like morphology, texture, margin and so on by application of machine learning. Further, feature selection is conducted to determine the most relevant features. The classification of a breast lesion as benign and malignant is carried out by implementing machine learning-based algorithms using different classifiers like a neural network, decision tree, support vector machine (SVM), and so on to automate BI-RADS criteria.

8.5   ISSUES AND CHALLENGES

The image classification techniques based on the existing machine learning approach have been used to classify biomedical images, mainly for the segmentation and classification of breast cancer images. There are different methods for segmentation and classification, but a robust approach is always a research problem. However, machine learning has some capability to address the issues of robustness. This can

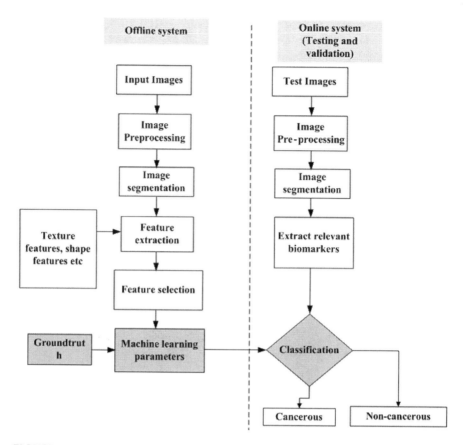

FIGURE 8.8   Block diagram of implementation of the machine learning approach.

be achieved by applying appropriate machine learning techniques in any or all stages of classification, such as feature extraction, feature selection, classification and detection. Deep learning overcomes this limitation with the use of convolutional neural networks (CNNs), which make use of the reconstructed images as input, and the processing is done via various layers [41]. Further, the probabilistic prediction is performed using machine learning methods whose inputs are the image features of the segmented images. Although research and studies on breast cancer diagnosis are numerous in the literature, a robust approach can be developed that can deal with different types of modalities and patients of different age groups. Most importantly, the cancer detection will be able to take place at early stages so that the lives of many can be saved [43].

Classifiers using machine learning techniques depend on feature extraction methods as to what types of features are extracted and subjected for classification. The image information in the form of structural and statistical features plays an important role in assessment of performance of the classification methods [43]. Deep learning has proved to be a promising machine learning approach recently in the area of medical imaging and also breast cancer detection. This network can handle a large amount of data and can process it using a higher number of hidden layers as compared to a conventional neural network [41]. There are a number of variants of the deep neural network such as the convolutional neural network (CNN), the recurrent neural network (RNN) and so on, which are used in different types of applications based on the requirements of learning categories.

8.6 CONCLUSION

Breast cancer is reported as the second leading cause of death in women globally, and its impact is significant in Asian countries. Due to a lack of clinical expertise, CAD plays an important role in assisting physicians and radiologists to effectively diagnose breast cancer cases. In this chapter, we have discussed the background of breast cancer detection, a number of breast imaging modalities which are used for diagnosis, and the role of machine learning. A comparison of all modalities has been made and mammograms are reported as the most commonly used in all cases of breast cancer treatment and diagnosis after detection of cancerous tissues inside breast images. Machine learning and AI techniques with signal processing tools have greatly helped improve the performance in CAD and in diagnosis results of breast cancer. The emergence of deep learning as the most powerful machine learning method has also been discussed.

LEARNING OUTCOMES

After studying this chapter, the students and learners will be able to:

- Explain the severity of breast cancer among women
- Implement a CAD system if having some knowledge of machine learning
- Enumerate breast image modalities
- Explain the performance measures of CAD for breast cancer diagnosis

EXERCISE FOR PRACTICE AND DISCUSSION

1. What is the best diagnostic tool used in breast cancer detection?
2. How can we detect breast cancer at an early stage? Will the machine learning method play any role in early detection?
3. Cancer in breast images of older women can be detected more easily as compared to young women. Explain this statement.
4. After the detection of cancer, the determination of the stage of cancer is very important. Discuss how we can assess at what stage the breast cancer is present in mammograms or any other medical image modalities.
5. Suggest few parameters which are used to measure the dimension of cancerous regions inside breast images.

REFERENCES

1. Veronesi, U., Goldhirsch, A., Veronesi, P., Gentilini, O. D., & Leonardi, M. C. (Eds.). (2017). *Breast cancer: Innovations in research and management*. Springer.

2. American Cancer Society. (2019). Breast Cancer Facts & Figures 2019–2020. Atlanta: American Cancer Society, Inc. 2019. www.cancer.org/content/dam/cancer-org/research/cancer-facts-and-statistics/breast-cancer-facts-and-figures/breast-cancer-facts-and-figures-2019-2020.pdf

3. Siegel, R. L., Miller, K. D., & Jemal, A. (2020). Cancer statistics, 2020. *CA: A cancer Journal for Clinicians, 70*(1), 7–30.

4. Jaglan, P., Dass, R., & Duhan, M. (2019). Breast cancer detection techniques: Issues and challenges. *Journal of the Institution of Engineers (India): Series B*, 1–8.

5. Yilmaz, R. (2019). Breast imaging. In Marina Alvarez Benito & Julia Campes Herroro (Eds.), *Breast cancer* (pp. 189–222). Springer.

6. Heath, Michael, Bowyer, Kevin, Kopans, Daniel, Moore, Richard, & Kegelmeyer, W. Philip. (2001). The Digital Database for Screening Mammography. In M. J. Yaffe (Ed.), *Proceedings of the Fifth International Workshop on Digital Mammography* (pp. 212–218). Medical Physics Publishing.

7. Heath, Michael, Bowyer, Kevin, Kopans, Daniel, Moore, Richard, Kegelmeyer, W. Philip, Chang, Kyong, & Munish Kumaran, S. (1998). Current status of the Digital Database for Screening Mammography. In N. Karssemeijer, M. Thijssen, J. Hendriks, & L. van Erning (Eds.), *Digital mammography: Computational imaging and vision* (Vol. 13, pp. 457–460). Springer. https://doi.org/10.1007/978-94-011-5318-8_75

8. Yassin, N. I., Omran, S., El Houby, E. M., & Allam, H. (2018). Machine learning techniques for breast cancer computer aided diagnosis using different image modalities: A systematic review. *Computer Methods and Programs in Biomedicine, 156*, 25–45.

9. Dheeba, J., Singh, N. A., & Selvi, S. T. (2014). Computer-aided detection of breast cancer on mammograms: A swarm intelligence optimized wavelet neural network approach. *Journal of Biomedical Informatics, 49*, 45–52.

10. Singh, S. P., & Urooj, S. (2016). An improved CAD system for breast cancer diagnosis based on generalized pseudo-Zernike moment and Ada-DEWNN classifier. *Journal of Medical Systems, 40*(4), 105. https://link.springer.com/article/10.1007%2Fs10916-016-0454-0

11. Hariraj, V., Khairunizam, W., Ibrahim, Z., Shahriman, A. B., Razlan, Z. M., Rajendran, T., & Sathiyasheelan, R. (2018). Fuzzy multi-layer SVM classification of breast cancer mammogram images. *International Journal of Mechanical Engineering and Technology, 9*(8), 1281–1299.

12. El-Sokary, N., Arafa, A. A., Asad, A. H., & Hefny, H. A. (2019). Computer-aided detection system for breast cancer based on GMM and SVM. *Arab Journal of Nuclear Sciences and Applications, 52*(2), 142–150.

13. Alqudah, A. M., Algharib, H. M., Algharib, A. M., & Algharib, H. M. (2019). Computer aided diagnosis system for automatic two stages classification of breast mass in digital mammogram images. *Biomedical Engineering: Applications, Basis and Communications, 31*(1), 1950007.

14. Singh, B. K., Jain, P., Banchhor, S. K., & Verma, K. (2019). Performance evaluation of breast lesion detection systems with expert delineations: A comparative investigation on mammographic images. *Multimedia Tools and Applications, 78*(16), 22421–22444.

15. Vanderheyden, B., & Xie, Y. (2020). Mammography image BI-RADS classification using OHPLall. *2020 IEEE Sixth International Conference on Big Data Computing*

Service and Applications (BigDataService) (pp. 120–127). IEEE. https://doi.org/ 10.1109/BigDataService49289.2020.00026.

16. Lee, H., & Chen, Y. P. P. (2015). Image based computer aided diagnosis system for cancer detection. *Expert Systems with Applications, 42*(12), 5356–5365.

17. Al-Dhabyani, W., Gomaa, M., Khaled, H., & Fahmy, A. (2020). Dataset of breast ultrasound images. *Data in Brief, 28*, 104863.

18. Abdelwahed, N. M., Eltoukhy, M. M., & Wahed, M. E. (2015). Computer aided system for breast cancer diagnosis in ultrasound images. *Journal of Ecology of Health & Environment, 3*(3), 71–76.

19. Flores, W. G., de Albuquerque Pereira, W. C., & Infantosi, A. F. C. (2015). Improving classification performance of breast lesions on ultrasonography. *Pattern Recognition, 48*(4), 1125–1136.

20. Menon, R. V., Raha, P., Kothari, S., Chakraborty, S., Chakrabarti, I., & Karim, R. (2015, December). Automated detection and classification of mass from breast ultrasound images. *2015 Fifth National Conference on Computer Vision, Pattern Recognition, Image Processing and Graphics (NCVPRIPG)* (pp. 1–4). IEEE. https:// doi.org/10.1109/NCVPRIPG.2015.7490070

21. Xian, M., Zhang, Y., & Cheng, H. D. (2015). Fully automatic segmentation of breast ultrasound images based on breast characteristics in space and frequency domains. *Pattern Recognition, 48*(2), 485–497.

22. Gu, P., Lee, W. M., Roubidoux, M. A., Yuan, J., Wang, X., & Carson, P. L. (2016). Automated 3D ultrasound image segmentation to aid breast cancer image interpretation. *Ultrasonics, 65*, 51–58.

23. Shan, J., Alam, S. K., Garra, B., Zhang, Y., & Ahmed, T. (2016). Computer-aided diagnosis for breast ultrasound using computerized BI-RADS features and machine learning methods. *Ultrasound in Medicine & Biology, 42*(4), 980–988.

24. Singh, B. K., Verma, K., & Thoke, A. S. (2016). Fuzzy cluster based neural network classifier for classifying breast tumours in ultrasound images. *Expert Systems with Applications, 66*, 114–123.

25. Singh, B. K., Verma, K., Thoke, A. S., & Suri, J. S. (2017). Risk stratification of 2D ultrasound-based breast lesions using hybrid feature selection in machine learning paradigm. *Measurement, 105*, 146–157.

26. Luo, Y., Liu, L., Huang, Q., & Li, X. (2017). A novel segmentation approach combining region-and edge-based information for ultrasound images. *BioMed Research International, 2017*, 89157341.

27. Liu, L., Li, K., Qin, W., Wen, T., Li, L., Wu, J., & Gu, J. (2018). Automated breast tumour detection and segmentation with a novel computational framework of whole ultrasound images. *Medical & Biological Engineering & Computing, 56*(2), 183–199.

28. Uzunhisarcikli, E., & Goreke, V. (2018). A novel classifier model for mass classification using BI-RADS category in ultrasound images based on Type-2 fuzzy inference system. *Sādhanā, 43*(9), 1–12, www.ias.ac.in/article/fulltext/sadh/043/09/0138; https://doi.org/10.1007/s12046-018-0915-x

29. Daoud, M. I., Atallah, A. A., Awwad, F., Al-Najjar, M., & Alazrai, R. (2019). Automatic superpixel-based segmentation method for breast ultrasound images. *Expert Systems with Applications, 121*, 78–96.

30. Panigrahi, L., Verma, K., & Singh, B. K. (2019). Ultrasound image segmentation using a novel multi-scale Gaussian kernel fuzzy clustering and multi-scale vector field convolution. *Expert Systems with Applications, 115*, 486–498.

31. Kozegar, E., Soryani, M., Behnam, H., Salamati, M., & Tan, T. (2019). Computer aided detection in automated 3-D breast ultrasound images: A survey. *Artificial Intelligence Review*, 1–23.

32. Virmani, J., & Agarwal, R. (2019). Effect of despeckle filtering on classification of breast tumours using ultrasound images. *Biocybernetics and Biomedical Engineering, 39*(2), 536–560.

33. Lyu, S., & Wang, J. (2019). Computer aided diagnosis of breast cancer based on ultrasound image. *Investigación Clínica, 60*(2), 546–554.

34. Xu, Y., Wang, Y., Yuan, J., Cheng, Q., Wang, X., & Carson, P. L. (2019). Medical breast ultrasound image segmentation by machine learning. *Ultrasonics, 91*, 1–9.

35. Chang, Y. W., Chen, Y. R., Ko, C. C., Lin, W. Y., & Lin, K. P. (2020). A novel computer-aided-diagnosis system for breast ultrasound images based on BI-RADS categories. *Applied Sciences, 10*(5), 1830.

36. Kuhl, C. K., Strobel, K., Bieling, H., Leutner, C., Schild, H. H., & Schrading, S. (2017). Supplemental breast MR imaging screening of women with average risk of breast cancer. *Radiology, 283*(2), 361–370.

37. Dalmiş, M. U., Vreemann, S., Kooi, T., Mann, R. M., Karssemeijer, N., & Gubern-Mérida, A. (2018). Fully automated detection of breast cancer in screening MRI using convolutional neural networks. *Journal of Medical Imaging* (Bellingham), *5*(1), 014502. https://doi.rog/10.1117/1.JMI.5.1.014502.

38. Venkata, M. D., & Lingamgunta, S. (2019) Triple-modality breast cancer diagnosis and analysis in middle aged women by logistic regression. *International Journal of Innovative Technology and Exploring Engineering, 8*(4), 2278–3075.

39. Herent, P., Schmauch, B., Jehanno, P., Dehaene, O., Saillard, C., Balleyguier, C., Arfi-Rouche, J., & Jégou, S. (2019). Detection and characterization of MRI breast lesions using deep learning. *Diagnostic and Interventional Imaging, 100*(4), 219–225.

40. Spak, D. A., Plaxco, J. S., Santiago, L., Dryden, M. J., & Dogan, B. E. (2017). BI-RADS® fifth edition: A summary of changes. *Diagnostic and Interventional Imaging, 98*(3), 179–190.

41. Tagliafico, A. S., Piana, M., Schenone, D., Lai, R., Massone, A. M., & Houssami, N. (2020). Overview of radiomics in breast cancer diagnosis and prognostication. *The Breast, 49*, 74–80.

42. Gong, S., Liu, C., Ji, Y., Zhong, B., Li, Y., & Dong, H. (2019). Image and video understanding based on deep learning. In *Advanced image and video processing using MATLAB* (pp. 513–553). Springer.

43. Nahid, A. A., & Kong, Y. (2017). Involvement of machine learning for breast cancer image classification: A survey. *Computational and Mathematical Methods in Medicine, 2017*, 3781951.

9 Sickle Cell Disease Management
A Machine Learning Approach

LEARNING OBJECTIVES

After reading this chapter, students will learn:

- Overview of sickle cell disease (SCD)
- Two main approaches of treatment of SCD patients
- Importance of ML- and AI-based models for SCD diagnosis
- Management of SCD using ML-based model

In this chapter, a machine learning model-based case study for sickle cell disease (SCD) management is discussed. The management system model discussed in this chapter is divided into five parts. The first part discusses the disease, its complications, its footprint across the world and its medication. Discussion in the second part is based on the machine learning approach for predicting the severity of sickle cell disease in patients based on their pathological attributes and clinical complications. Here the application of the machine learning approach is discussed to predict the number of clinical complications of an individual patient, and this predicted count is considered an indicator of the severity of the disease in the patient. The third and the fourth part under the discussion of this management model are based on accurate prediction of the amount of dosage of hydroxyurea (HU) for treatment and classification of the patient's response to the dosage respectively. The fifth part of this chapter is directed towards the application of machine learning approaches to provide a complete SCD management system which will assist clinicians in the treatment of SCD patients, especially in rural areas.

9.1 INTRODUCTION

Sickle cell anaemia is seen as a common genetic disease in some communities in a few states of India. The disease is reported as a most common and serious blood-related disorder which is considered a genetic disorder. Sickle cell disease (SCD) seriously affects the quality of life and life expectancy of persons if they do not follow strict advice and precautions. Various research organizations and medical institutions report the presence of SCD cases in the states of Chhattisgarh, Maharashtra, Gujrat,

DOI: 10.1201/9781003097808-9

Kerala and a few others. There is sufficient evidence observed in these states related to SCD cases, and the subsequent analysis also suggests that the presence of SCD can be found in many other states in the country. In fact, the sickle cell institute in Chhattisgarh state, located at Raipur, has brought out a handbook on SCD [1] that highlights that affected persons carry the traits or disease. SCD poses challenges and a threat to life. Whereas the traits do not cause the potential for death, persons having the traits need to follow a disciplined life and take precautions. SCD or its traits are actually seen as a prototype whose consequences may range from illness to serious illness and also death in a few cases [2]. As reported by the World Health Organization (WHO) regarding SCD, almost 5% of the total population are carriers of SCD traits or even affected by the disease, and the percentage goes up to 25% in a few areas of the world. So, SCD is not only a threat in few states of India but all across the globe [3], especially in the African population where SCD is seen as a common genetic disease, and the disease is regarded as a serious threat in the form of thalassemia in Middle Eastern and Asian countries.

The haemoglobin is imbalanced in SCD cases when the content of the haemoglobin is checked, especially in the red blood cells of the patients. The unusual haemoglobin amount is the main reason for SCD and such a situation is called sickle haemoglobin (HbS). Due to this sickle cell disease, the haemoglobin and the shape of the red blood cell are adversely affected and the body of the SCD person begins when sickle (crescent)-shaped red blood cells are produced [1]. Due to the rigid structure and shape of the red blood cells, and the unusual shape and rigid surface of the red blood cells, these persons are affected by anaemia [2]. The flow of abnormal red blood cells is reported which is blocked from blood vessels, and this causes serious consequences such as extreme abdominal pain, crises and so on, and this may further cause damage to some vital organs of the body. In SCD patients, there can be some other clinical complications such as anaemia, jaundice, icterus, pneumonia, repeated blood transfusions, shortening of limb and so on, and therefore it becomes important that timely and effective treatments are provided to SCD-affected people. The proper treatment of SCD disorder will help patients to lead a quality and healthy life, and life expectancy is also improved. Research-based findings suggest that the conventional practices of diagnosis and treatment of SCD are not appropriate, and it requires early diagnosis using CAD-based systems so that effective and early detection and then diagnosis can be facilitated for patients. A robust patient care system and effective and planned treatment are much-needed measures for SCD-affected persons.

Generally, two methods for treating SCD patients are reported. The first method is carrying out bone marrow transplantation, and the second method is the medication hydroxyurea. In the former approach to treatment, the aim is to cure serious complications in older patients, and the approach appears to be very promising for the treatment of sickle cell anaemia and disease in people in younger age groups too, whereas the second method helps reduce the complications due to SCD and an appropriate amount of fetal haemoglobin (HbF) is produced. A fraction of sickle haemoglobin is reduced in red blood cells (RBC) that helps maintain the dosage of hydroxyurea accurately [3]. Despite these methods being widely used, there are still some serious issues and challenges with the methods. There is an adequate amount of risk associated with bone marrow transplantation and finding a donor for bone marrow is also a challenging task involved in this method of cure. In the other method of treatment, the medication hydroxyurea, proper dosage control is needed for the patient and guidance of a healthcare expert is strictly required for avoiding the possibility of infection due improper dosage. Due to minimum risk in patients, the treatment of SCD patients is done by the expert healthcare professionals using the hydroxyurea medication. Based on reports by the US Food and Drug Administration (FDA), hydroxyurea is approved as a suitable drug for reducing painful episodes from the disease. A study in [9] reports that the painful episodes for SCD patients are significantly reduced with the appropriate dosage of hydroxyurea, with an up to 50% reduction.

The biggest difficulty in disease management of SCD patients is in exploring the huge amount of data, which is time-consuming and involves risks related to observational errors. The expertise of medical professionals and their experience determine the quality of treatment, and due to this fact, a lot of data analysis takes place on patients suffering from SCD. In the last two decades, intelligent CAD systems have been developed to assist physicians and clinicians in the prediction of the severity of SCD in patients. The CAD system is used to predict the appropriate amount of dosage of hydroxyurea that helps in reducing the painful episodes and clinical complications are lessened. Then, the determination of dosage becomes easier if the patient responds to the amount of dosage of hydroxyurea or not. The very first study on this area using an AI-based treatment and management system for SCD, was seen in the year 2000 [10], that employed machine learning (ML) methods for the prediction of response of patients to doses of hydroxyurea. Later, many other researchers applied different machine learning models to predict the severity of crises, to predict dosage, and for other crucial outcomes for disease management, which is explained in the next section of this chapter including the first one.

Organization of this chapter is as follows: the current Section 9.1, of this chapter gives an introduction to sickle cell disease, its treatment, management and the requirements of machine learning. In Section 9.2, studies based on the application of machine learning models to predict the severity of sickle cell disease in a patient are discussed. Section 9.3 of this chapter gives a detailed explanation of different machine learning models used in the past two decades to predict an adequate amount of dosage. Section 9.4 of this chapter discusses the prediction of a patient's response to medication using machine learning models and pathological attributes. Section 9.5 proposes a sickle cell disease management model, which is a combination of the models discussed in Sections 9.2, 9.3 and 9.4. Section 9.5 of the chapter tries to provide a complete management model for the sickle cell patient to assist clinicians. In the last section, section 9.6 gives a conclusion note of this chapter.

9.2   SEVERITY DETECTION OF SICKLE CELL DISEASE

Based on the available literature, the machine learning approach for severity detection in the SCD patient was applied to patient-specific data in one of the following ways:

9.2.1 Analysis of Clinical Complications

Clinical complications such as icterus, cyanosis, lymphadenopathy, haemolytic face, bony tenderness, shortening limb, short stature, acute chest syndrome, acute pain crises, chronic pain, delayed growth, eye problems, gallstones and so on, along with pathological information such as percentage sickle haemoglobin, are essential features in predicting severity of SCD patients. Many of the available statistical study-based literatures provided evidence of a statistical association between clinical outcomes and pathological information. In one study [4], the authors evaluated haematological parameters (PCV and WBC) as an important indicator of SCD-related clinical outcome. More than 100 persons were involved in this study, which showed stable SCD indicators. In this study, significance statistics were observed between haematological parameters of persons and number of complications that were related to stroke, crisis, cholelithiasis, acute chest syndrome, nephropathy, priapism, avascular necrosis of head of femur, leg ulcer and blindness. The chi-square test was applied in order to compare various frequencies and also to generate the p-values. The study and its results indicate that the complications related to SCD are very much associated with increased WBC counts for p-value 0.03. It was also reported that a closed association was seen between increase in WBC count and complications with p-value 0.07. This study also highlights that the prediction of SCD outcomes can be made with the help of WBC counts.

Another statistical analysis-based study was recently reported by [5]. The study was conducted to test the statistical significance between haemoglobin variants and the number of clinical complications associated with SCD patients, and also between individual complications and haemoglobin variants. Seven clinical complications such as cyanosis, lymphadenopathy, icterus and so on, and three haemoglobin variants: haemoglobin (HbS), fetal haemoglobin (HbF), and adult haemoglobin (HbA), were considered in the study. The study was conducted with 827 individuals with SCD, and the tests applied in the study were Spearman's correlation test and the Mann–Whitney U test. Reported results verified the statistical association between clinical complications and the severity with haemoglobin variants.

9.2.2 Analysis of Clinical Attributes

In [6], the authors demonstrated how machine learning can be applied to predict a severity crisis in individual SCD patients. In the above-mentioned article, the outcome of the machine learning predictive model was random variable Y with two possible values as 'mild' and 'severe'. The response of the machine learning model is based on input clinical attributes X. The experiment was performed on a children dataset with 42 samples. Each sample consisted of 15 different clinical attributes as input features for the model. Features used in the model are leucocyte count, neutrophile count, platelets count and so on. The severity crisis is based on levels of haemoglobin, so the thresholding was applied on haemoglobin for a binary class. A haemoglobin level of more than 4g/dl was considered 'mild' and less than 4g/dl was considered 'severe'. Haemoglobin was not included as an input feature for the training and testing of the machine learning model. The complete dataset was divided into two parts: the first one was training data and the second one was testing data.

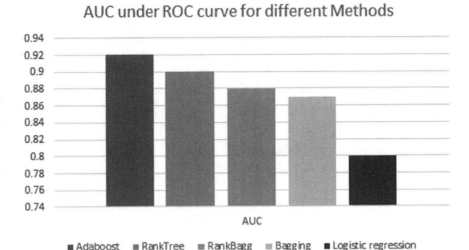

FIGURE 9.1 ROC curve for different methods.

A supervised machine learning approach using **R** software package was applied. The authors had explored Adaboost, Ranktree, Rankbagg, Bagging and logistic regression methods for severity prediction and identification of significant biomarkers for severity prediction. Figure 9.1 represents the area under the ROC curve (AUC) for different methods applied in [6].

ADABOOST: This is a variational method in which an approximation $F(x)$ is repeatedly changed by adding small corrections to it, given by the weak prediction functions. The four most important variables were identified by ranking the variables. The area under a ROC curve (AUC) obtained is 92%, which confirms that Adaboost gives the best prediction of severity of an SCD patient.

Bagging: Classification using bagging shows a low value of AUC in a ROC curve, that is, 87%; however, among the top four dominant features for the classification model, two features are the same as in the Adaboost model.

Rank Tree: The algorithm is based on building a binary tree-structured scoring function. The AUC obtained under a ROC curve was 90%. However, it was less than the Adaboost method but better than other models explored in the article.

RankBagg: The area under the ROC curve for this method was 88%, which shows mediocre performance.

Logistic regression: The mathematical model used in logistic regression is given by

$$\log \frac{P\left(Y = \dfrac{1}{X}\right)}{1 - P\left(Y = \dfrac{1}{X}\right)} = \alpha + \beta X. \tag{9.1}$$

Here in Equation (9.1), X denotes the set of input features and Y indicates the set of output class. Starting with a null model stepwise selection procedure, an auxiliary variable is added with the most significant score statistic, and the process terminates when there are no more variables available for addition into the model. The logistic regression shows the least value of AUC in a ROC curve, that is, 80%.

9.2.3 ANALYSIS OF MICROSCOPIC IMAGES OF RBC

Article [7] confirms that RBCs in sickle cell anaemia are correlated with the severity of the clinical disease. Hence, the analysis of the morphology of a microscopic image of red blood cells by applying image processing and machine learning techniques can be used to predict the dominance of abnormal RBCs. In several research articles, detection, classification and the counting of different shapes of red blood cells were performed. Figure 9.2 shows a microscopic image of a red blood cell.

In a recent article [8], the counting of normal and abnormal red blood cells was performed. An image processing technique was employed on a single blood smear image and normal RBCs were identified and counted using two different methods. The first method is Circle Hough Transform (CHT), and the second one is Watershed Transform (WT).

Circle Hough Transform (CHT): This algorithm is based on detecting a circle in an image. However, before applying this method, the first few steps involve pre-processing, that is, image acquisition, RGB to grey conversion, noise filtering and edge detection, and after that CHT can be applied. CHT also consists of three essential steps. The first step is called accumulator array computation and foreground pixels having high gradient values are represented as candidates for testing among subjects, and considered as signing "votes" in the accumulator array. When implementing the CHT method, the candidate pixels are involved in the voting process across the patterns. This causes the appearance of a full circle of a particular radius. In the second step, the centre of the circle is estimated, and the third step is based on estimation of the radius.

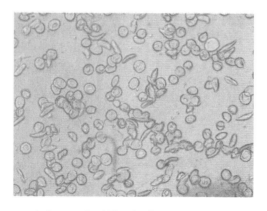

FIGURE 9.2   Microscopic image of red blood cell.

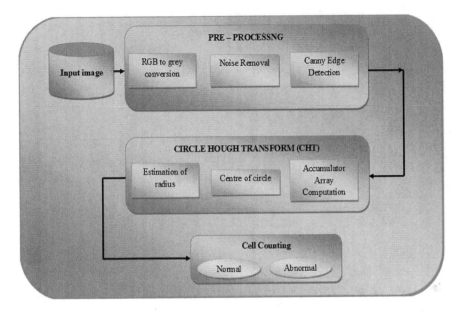

FIGURE 9.3   Circle Hough Transform method based normal and abnormal cell counting.

Figure 9.3 shows the CHT algorithm steps applied for counting individual cells. The total count of the cells was 233 and the CHT algorithm detected 138 cells as normal and 95 cells as abnormal.

Watershed Transform (WT): This method performs well for segmentation. The method is applied on a gradient image rather than a raw image. The marking of foreground objects and background locations of the basis of the method. Important steps used in watershed based segmentation are shown in Figure 9.4 [9]. The effect factor is computed as:

$$Effect\ Factor = 4 \times \pi \times area\ /\ Perimeter^2. \qquad (9.2)$$

In WT, the algorithm effect factor was calculated based on Equation (9.2). The cells are classified based on the value of this effect factor. For normal cells, the effect factor is around 0.9. Watershed segmentation counted 123 cells as normal and the remaining 110 cells as abnormal. The counting efficiency and processing time for the CHT method is better than for the WT method.

There is a broad scope of research on a hybrid model combining machine learning on pathological attributes with microscopic images for severity prediction disease at an early stage. This will help clinicians in treatment planning.

9.3   HYDROXYUREA DOSAGE PREDICTION FOR SCD PATIENTS

Abnormal RBCs are responsible for causing obstruction or blockage in the smooth flow of blood through blood vessels of the body. Consequently, some serious

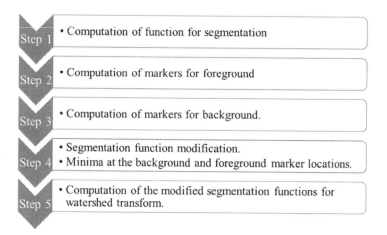

Step 1 • Computation of function for segmentation

Step 2 • Computation of markers for foreground

Step 3 • Computation of markers for background.

Step 4 • Segmentation function modification.
• Minima at the background and foreground marker locations.

Step 5 • Computation of the modified segmentation functions for watershed transform.

FIGURE 9.4   Essential steps for Watershed segmentation.

complications can result such as anaemia, repeated blood transfusions, icterus, jaundice, pneumonia, shortening limb and so on. Given such complications, it becomes essential to provide timely and effective treatment for SCD-affected patients so that increased life expectancy and quality of life can be achieved among patients with SCD diseases. Recent studies and research suggest that the treatment of SCD patients requires special care and AI-based diagnosis systems. The existing approaches to treatment by the clinicians and physicians involved need to be replaced by an expert CAD system for diagnosis so that SCD symptoms are detected at an early stage. The patient care model and treatment method using CAD-based diagnosis is reported, and two well-known methods are used, bone marrow transplantation and the medication hydroxyurea (HU). There are some serious complications for older patients with the bone marrow transplantation method, whereas for a younger age group, the approach shows good results in curing sickle cell anaemia. The medication HU assists in reducing the complications, and foetal haemoglobin (HbF) is created that further helps in achieving a reduced amount of sickle haemoglobin in (RBCs) [3]. There are both advantages and disadvantages associated with both approaches to treatment. Healthcare professionals and their expertise are involved in assisting with and maintaining proper dosages of HU for the treatment of SCD.

Both approaches to treating SCD patients have their positive and negative outcomes. For instance, bone marrow transplantation is a risky procedure and it requires a bone marrow donor, whereas for treatment through HU, an accurate amount of dosage under the guidance of a clinical expert is required since improper dosage of HU can have certain complications

Data exploration is needed to handle with the huge amount of data for managing the effective treatment of SCD patients. The observational error changes due to the huge data and using manual approach of the treatment, the expertise and experience of the professional determines the quality of the treatment and its impact. The importance of an automated model of treatment for the disease management of SCD patients lies in the prediction of an appropriate dosage of hydroxyurea.

ML-based models and CAD systems are used to analyse the data related to SCD patients, which also reduces the burden on healthcare professionals. The AI models predict the accurate quantum amount of dosage of HU in milligrams. In the ML-based approaches reported in research and studies, a number of ML-based classifiers were developed and tested in datasets of SCD patients. This dataset in the study [3], included 1,168 subjects and the database was applied for ML models having 13 attributes as input clinical features, aimed at obtaining a target value of the appropriate value of HU dosage in mg. The dataset created in the work includes different groups: 70% for training, 10% for validation and the remaining 20% for final testing and for estimating the performance of the classification model. The dosage of HU was divided into three bins with equal class size. The overall dataset was divided into three different groups: 70% for training, 10% for validation and the remaining 20% for final testing and for estimating the performance of the classification model. Eight different ML models were developed and tested by the authors, and they are the Elman Neural Network (ENN) with 30 hidden layers; the Jordan Neural Network (JNN) with 30 hidden layers; the Elman-Jordan Hybrid Neural Network (EJNN) with 30 hidden layers; the multilayer perceptron, trained using the Levenberg-Marquardt algorithm (LEVNN) with 2 hidden layers; the Random Forest Classifier (RFC) with 200 trees; the Support Vector Machine (SVM); the Linear Combiner Network (LNN); and the Random Oracle Model (ROM). The models were evaluated based on seven performance measures: classification accuracy, sensitivity, specificity, Youden's J statistic (J Score), precision, area under ROC curve (AUC), and F1 scores. The reported results confirm the accurate prediction of HU dosage can be made with the help of ML-based treatment and diagnosis models. The performance measures are used for all the classifiers and related models. The overall performance of the Levenberg-Marquardt learning method for LEVNN and RFC classifiers is found to be better as compared to other ML and non-ML models. The dosage of hydroxyurea is maintained more than three bins, and thus the proposed system is realized in an efficient way.

Recent research in the field of medicine for SCD patients [10] applied two machine learning models for prediction of dosage and compared the performance of both models. The experimental set-up for the objective is shown in Figure 9.5.

Input dataset: The dataset used in the study consist of 12 input attributes and one output target. The input attributes are the predictors for ML models and they are listed in Table 9.1. The target variable includes HU dosages, and the output target variables are dosage of HU that is further classified into high, mild and moderate dosages. In this study, the number of subjects in the dataset were 1,128.

Data division: For training and testing, the dataset is divided into two groups: training and testing. Holdout data division protocol was used with 75% data for training and 25% data for testing.

Classification model: Two classification models named: Long Short-Term Memory networks (LSTM) and Extreme learning machines (ELM) were used for dosage prediction, and five performance measures named: classification accuracy, sensitivity, specificity, precision and F1 score, were calculated for comparison of the performance of the two models. The calculated performance metric of the two models is shown in Table 9.2.

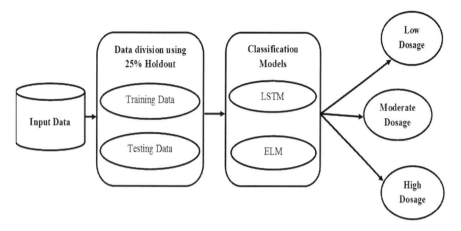

FIGURE 9.5   Experimental set-up for dosage prediction.

TABLE 9.1
Clinical Attributes as Input Features

No	Clinical Attribute
1	Weight of patient (in kg)
2	Aspartate Aminotransferase (AST)
3	Mean Corpuscular Volume (MCV)
4	Bilirubin (BILI)
5	Neutrophils (white blood cell)
6	Fetal Haemoglobin (HbF)
7	Haemoglobin (Hb)
8	Alanine aminotransferase (ALT)
9	Reticulocyte Count (RETIC A)
10	Platelets (PLTS)
11	Lactate dehydrogenase (LDH)
12	Reticulocyte Count (RETIC %)

LSTM: LSTM is a special type of recurrent neural network (RNN) with feedback connections. A five-layer deep network using LSTM was designed and applied in the afore-mentioned dataset, as shown in Figure 9.6. The deep network model applied consisted of 100 hidden layers; tanh function was used for activation; and for gate activation, the sigmoid function was applied. The results shown in the study, as depicted in Table 9.2, confirm that the class-wise accuracy of LSTM is around 78% for each class and also as per the values of performance measures, LSTM performs better than ELM. However, in terms of training time, the performance of LSTM is poor.

TABLE 9.2
LSTM and ELM Performance Comparison

	Class 1		Class 2		Class 3	
	ELM	**LSTM**	**ELM**	**LSTM**	**ELM**	**LSTM**
Accuracy	0.52	0.78	0.52	0.78	0.52	0.78
Sensitivity	0.10	0.55	0.04	0.55	0.81	0.77
Specificity	0.91	0.89	0.89	0.93	0.15	0.79
Precision	0.48	0.72	0.23	0.82	0.56	0.79
F1 Score	0.16	0.62	0.07	0.66	0.66	0.78

ELM: The extreme learning machine was first suggested [11] as a feedforward neural network with only one hidden layer. After some modification, it was modified to a network which is like a non-neuron network. The main feature of ELM networks is their training time, which is much less. Also, the tuning for the hidden layer is not required for ELM networks. The output function of ELM $f_L(x)f_L(x)$ is given by

$$f_L(x) = h(x)\beta \; f_L(x) = h(x)^2, \tag{9.3}$$

where

$$\beta = \begin{bmatrix} \beta_1 \\ \beta_2 \\ \beta_3 \\ \vdots \\ \beta_L \end{bmatrix} \text{and } h(x) = \begin{bmatrix} h_1(x) & h_2(x) & h_3(x) & h_l(x) \end{bmatrix}.$$

Here, β is used to denote a column matrix, each element of which represents the weights between the hidden layer and the output node; L denotes the number of nodes in the hidden layer; h(x) indicates row matrix, of which each element is seen as the output of the hidden layer for the input x; and the value of h(x) indicates a function for mapping n-dimensional input space to L-dimensional hidden-layer feature space. In this study, discussion was made for single-dimension data of the input. The performance of the ELM approach was found inferior to the LSTM network in terms of sensitivity, accuracy, precision, specificity and F1 score. The most salient feature of ELM lies in the manageable amount of training time, and the network is found to be faster than the LSTM network.

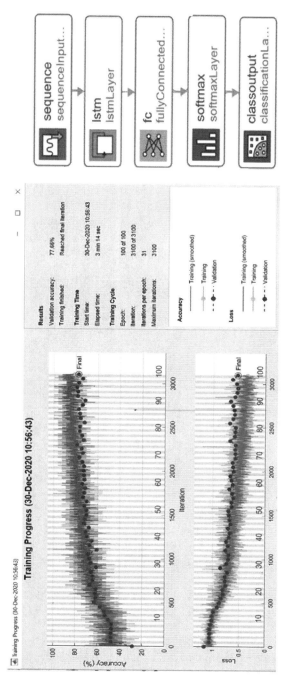

FIGURE 9.6 Experimental set-up and result for LSTM model.

9.4   PATIENT RESPONSE TO MEDICATIONS THROUGH HYDROXYUREA (HU)

Since the 1980s hydroxyurea (HU) medication has been prescribed by doctors for SCD patients. However, in 1998 it was finally approved by the US Food and Drug Administration (FDA) for treatment of adults with SCD, and for children with SCD it was approved by FDA in 2017. HU dosage reduces the complications and severity for SCD patients. It is also effective in reducing episodes of chest syndrome, blood transfusion and hospitalization.

> **Cole's Story***
>
> "This was my first activity without pain in years." Before Cole started taking hydroxyurea, she had frequent pain crises. For a while, she was in the hospital every few weeks. She wasn't able to keep a job. Then Cole's doctor recommended hydroxyurea. After she started taking it, Cole began to feel better. She even walked a 5K race just a few months later without going into crisis or having any pain. She was able to start working again and she has gone more than four years without a major pain crisis.

HU increases the count of fatal haemoglobin (HbF), which makes red blood cells bigger and it helps RBCs stay in a disc shape. HU dosage is strongly recommended by doctors for sickle cell anaemia patients, that is, sickle cell disease type SS (SCD-SS) and sickle beta zero (Sβ0) thalassemia. While taking medication through HU, patients are recommended to have a regular blood count check. The following observation are made by doctors:

(i) **Rise in haemoglobin levels:** HU dosage increases the total number of haemoglobins by creating new fatal haemoglobin (HbF). A rise in haemoglobin level after medication through HU is an indicator of a positive response in a patient.

(ii) **Rise in mean cell values (MCV):** HU dosage makes red blood cells bigger, which increases the MCV value in the test. A rise in the value of MCV after dosage of HU is also an indication of a positive response from the patient.

(iii) **Drop in neutrophil levels:** After medication with HU, the number of white blood cells goes down. However, it should not be too low. So, the dosage needs to be planned accordingly.

Based on the observations of these numbers and other clinical attributes, healthcare experts draw a conclusion that a patient is responding to the existing therapy or not. If they are not responding, then the expert makes changes in the therapy. After one or more follow-ups, the clinical expert again tries to identify the patient as responder or non-responder. This manual approach to identifying a patient as responder or non-responder needs lots of data exploration. For this reason, it is time-consuming and requires clinical expertise.

In the automated and computer-based model, ML approaches are applied by researchers in exploring the data during training and testing of the treatment involved in the diagnosis system of SCD patients. In one particular study [3], the respondents and their samples were classified using proposed models, and in the first study reported, AI methods were used for predicting the effect of hydroxyurea on patients suffering from SCD and sickle cell anaemia [12]. In the dataset used for the study, 23 clinical attributes were taken as input features that were subjected for learning and a single variable output is produced. The dataset included samples from 83 patients for predicting the HbF response by the SCD patients with the help of a traditional neural network approach. The prediction accuracy of 86.6% was obtained, whereas the linear regression model and correlation analysis failed to produce any correlation between HbF response of patients and 23 clinical attributes. However, the study was limited to a very small dataset of 83 patients, which raises a generalization ability-related question for the proposed model. The analysis in terms of specificity and sensitivity of the proposed model was not included as part of the study, and thus a robust performance classification could not be made. Additionally, the model appeared to be computationally very expensive because the data division protocol used was left out during the testing and training of the learning model.

In another important study on the classification model, reported in [13], the support vector machine (SVM) model is suggested for predicting the response of patients to HU dosage. The experiment was carried out in the study over a dataset of 304 patients having 18 attributes of persons involved in the study: sex, age, HbF, HbS, HbA2, Haematocrit, MCV, Hb, RDW, MCH, DLC (L, M, G), TLC, Plc, EnzSGOT and EnzSGPT. The sex of the subject is encoded as 1 for female and 2 for male candidates. The hydroxyurea value affects the attributes of patients after each visit and the response of the body changes accordingly. The HbF value is utilized for making the output classes standardized. The output class 1 (Responsive) indicates the HbF level in the patient, which was seen as high as 15, and class 0 (non-responsive) for an increase in the HbF level below the 20%. The experimental set-up of model is shown in Figure 9.7.

In the first stage, the feature selection technique was applied using WEKA software to find the rank of each feature. As shown in a block diagram, two approaches were applied for feature selection: (i) filter-based approach and (ii) wrapper-based approach. In the filter-based approach seven different methods named correlation ranking filter, gain ratio feature evaluator, information gain ranking filter, one-R feature evaluator, principal components, relief ranking filter and symmetrical uncertainty ranking filter were applied. Out of these seven methods, four of them considered the sickle haemoglobin (HbS) count before and after the dosage of HU is the most dominant feature. The other approach, that is, the wrapper-based approach, also shows that HbS is the most significant feature among all other available features. Based on a feature ranking list and with various data division protocol supports, a vector machine algorithm-based classification model was trained and tested. The model was tested with a different number of features as input predictors. The support vector machine (SVM)-based classification model classifies each instance as responder or non-responder. The performance of the classifier is assessed with calculated

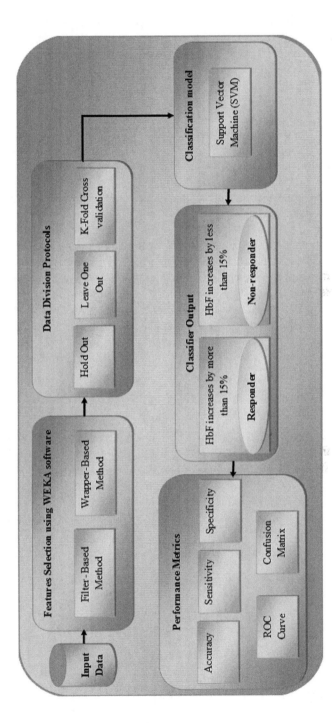

FIGURE 9.7   Experimental set-up for prediction of response for HU therapy.

performance metrics like: accuracy, sensitivity, specificity and so on. Based on the above results, authors suggested that the therapy response system performs best with: the Information Gain and OneR feature selection method using the hold-out classification method. The classification accuracy archived for the above-discussed model is 94%, and other measures like sensitivity and specificity were also more than 90%. However, the experiment was performed on a very small size of dataset. The model should be tested with a large dataset.

9.5   SCD MANAGEMENT PROPOSED MODEL

The proposed model, including three important sections for sickle cell disease management, is shown in Figure 9.8.

The proposed sickle cell disease management model consists of two different modes of input data. The first type of data includes pathological attributes such as haemoglobin levels, HbS, HbF, MCV and so on, and the second data consist of microscopic images of red blood cells for the same patients. In the feature set development section, the first step is to extract features from the images. Then the two sets of features are combined by data fusion, and after that, the relevant features need to be selected by applying feature selection tools. In the next stage, the developed feature set is applied to machine learning models for prediction of severity, accurate amount of dosage and the patient's response to the therapy. The proposed model will be helpful for clinicians for disease management. Also, it will mitigate the painful episodes, number of hospitalizations and severity crises in patients.

9.6   CONCLUSIONS

In the last few decades many researchers have applied various machine learning models in the clinical dataset of SCD patients. Some of them achieved very good results for prediction severity, medicine for SCD patients and their response to medication. These results helped clinicians in the effective treatment of disease. However, a complete sickle cell disease management model was missing, which is proposed in this chapter.

LEARNING OUTCOMES

After studying this chapter, students will be able to:

* Discuss SCD as a disease, its cause and consequences
* Explain the management of SCD and the role of ML-based methods

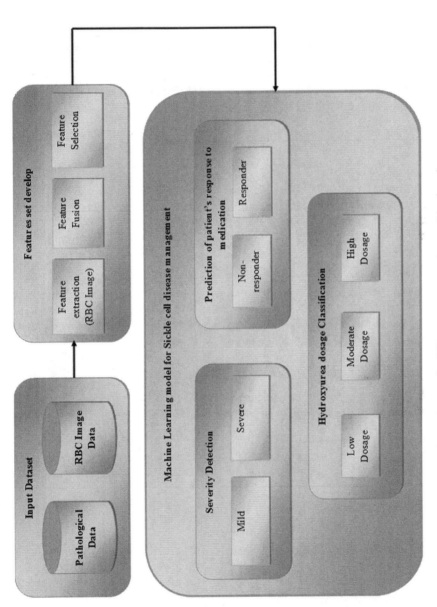

FIGURE 9.8 Proposed experimental set-up for SCD management using machine learning.

REFERENCES

1. Okpala, I. (2004). The intriguing contribution of white blood cells to sickle cell disease – A red cell disorder. *Blood Reviews, 18*(1), 65–73. https://doi.org/10.1016/s0268-960x(03)00037-7

2. Poillon, W. N., Kim, B. C. , & Castro, O. (1998). Intracellular hemoglobin S polymerization and the clinical severity of sickle cell anemia. *Blood, 91*(5), 1777–1783.

3. Khalaf, M. et al. (2017). Machine learning approaches to the application of disease modifying therapy for sickle cell using classification models. *Neurocomputing, 228*(C), 154–164. https://doi.org/10.1016/j.neucom.2016.10.043

4. Emmanuelchide, O., Charle, O., & Uchenna, O. (2011). Hematological parameters in association with outcomes in sickle cell anemia patients. *Indian Journal of Medical Sciences*, 65(9), 393–398. https://doi.org/10.4103/0019-5359.108955

5. Allayous, C., Clemencon, S., Diagne, B., & Emilion, R. (2008). Machine learning algorithms for predicting severe crises of sickle cell disease. *Mathematics Subject Classification*. https://idpoisson.fr/emilion/publ/MLASSC.pdf

6. Lonergan, G. J., Cline, D. B., & Abbondanzo, S. L. (2001). From the archives of the AFIP: Sickle cell anemia. *Radiographics, 21*(4), 971–994.

7. Abdulraheem Fadhel, M., Humaidi, A. J., & Oleiwi, S. R. (2017). Image processing-based diagnosis of sickle cell anemia in erythrocytes. In IEEE (Ed.), *2017 Annual Conference on New Trends in Information and Communications Technology Applications (NTICT)* (pp. 203–207). IEEE. https://doi.org/10.1109/NTICT.2017.7976124

8. *Proceedings of the International Conference on Soft Computing for Problem Solving, SocProS 2011* (Vol. 2). (Advances in Intelligent and Soft Computing). Springer India.

9. Candrilli, S. D., O'Brien, S. H., Ware, R. E., Nahata, M. C., Seiber, E. E., & Balkrishnan, R. (2011). Hydroxyurea adherence and associated outcomes among Medicaid enrollees with sickle cell disease. *American Journal of Hematology, 86*(3), 273–277. https://doi.org/10.1002/ajh.21968

10. Bin Huang, G., Zhou, H., Ding, X., & Zhang, R. (2012). Extreme learning machine for regression and multiclass classification. *IEEE Transactions on Systems, Man, and Cybernetics, Part B Cybernetics, 42*(2), 513–529.

11. Valafar, H. et al. (2000). Predicting the effectiveness of hydroxyurea in individual sickle cell anemia patients. *Artificial Intelligence in Medicine, 18*(2), 133–148.

12. Singh, B. K., Ojha, A., Bhoi, K. K., Bissoyi, A., & Patra, P. K. (2021). Prediction of hydroxyurea effect on sickle cell anemia patients using machine learning method. In A. A. Rizvanov, B, K. Singh, & P. Ganasala (Eds.), *Advances in Biomedical Engineering and Technology* (pp. 447–457). (Lecture Notes in Bioengineering). Springer. https://doi.org/10.1007/978-981-15-6329-4_37

10 Detection of Pulmonary Disease

LEARNING OBJECTIVES

The chapter aims to cover:

- Overview and types of pulmonary disorder
- Test and scanning methods used in analysis and diagnosis of the disorder
- Issues and challenges in diagnosis
- Application of machine learning in efficient disease diagnosis

Lung diseases are reported as common disease all over the world. It would not be enough to restrict the initial examination for a reliable diagnosis of these diseases. Pulmonary disease is associated with the lungs and can cause death if not detected at an early stage. Many such diseases have similar symptoms that cause difficulties in effective treatment, and this has led to further development in the analysis and detection of the disease. There are several methods such as electronic auscultations, imaging that uses X-rays and computed tomography (CT) scan for diagnosis of this disease. Data from the method can be used to improve diagnostic measures. Owing to electronic auscultation and various modern methods of signal and image processing analysis, it has become possible to obtain new diagnostic parameters. Machine learning is considered a suitable method for obtaining appropriate parameters by using suitable algorithms. Machine learning is used in many areas of medical imaging for medical diagnosis and treatment of various diseases. This chapter discusses the detection of pulmonary diseases.

10.1 INTRODUCTION TO PULMONARY DISORDERS

The lungs are the most vital organs for the proper functioning of a human body. The lungs help in inhaling and exhaling air and thus play an important role. The flow of blood inside the human body also depends on the functioning of the lungs.

Any improper or unusual behaviour in the functioning of the lungs is termed a pulmonary disorder [1]. There are three types of lung disorders, which are categorized as follows:

DOI: 10.1201/9781003097808-10

a. Airway Diseases – When the tubes which carry oxygen and other gases inside the body get narrowed or blocked, then airway diseases result [2]. The improper structure of the airway tubes allows very little space for gases to flow through them, which can cause the patient to feel as if they are breathing through a thin straw. Examples of airway disorders area asthma and chronic obstructive pulmonary disease.

b. Lung Tissue Disease – The occurrence of inflammation or swelling in the tissues of the lungs adversely affects the lung's structure. This causes a decrease in the ability of the lungs to expand, which has interferes with the function of the intake of oxygen and the release of carbon dioxide taking place properly. The patient suffering from this disease feels congestion in the chest as if the patient is wearing a very tight vest [3]. Examples of diseases in this category include sarcoidosis, pulmonary fibrosis and so on.

c. Lung Circulation Disease – Lung circulation diseases can cause clotting or inflammation in the air tubes. The blood vessels in the lungs get adversely affected, which causes a decrease in the ability to take up oxygen and release carbon dioxide [4]. Patients suffering from this disease should avoid exertion as at times they may feel short of breath. This disease is caused by abnormalities in blood vessels; therefore, it can also affect the function of the heart. The main example of this category is pulmonary hypertension.

10.2 RESTRICTIVE AND OBSTRUCTIVE LUNG DISEASES

Depending upon the conditions of the lung and its functions, pulmonary disorders are mainly categorized into two types:

a. Restrictive Lung disease
b. Obstructive Lung disease

Restrictive disease is further divided classified as: Intrinsic restrictive, Extrinsic restrictive and Neurological restrictive. Figure 10.1 shows various categories of restrictive and obstructive lung diseases.

10.2.1 OBSTRUCTIVE LUNG DISEASE

Obstructive lung diseases occur when the pulmonary airways get narrow. This affects a person's ability to completely exhale air from the lungs. Due to this narrowing of airways, every time a person breathes, some amount of air is left inside the lungs, which can cause obstruction [5]. A person suffering from obstructive lung disease may feel short of breath during heavy exercise or at times of exertion because the breathing rate increases heavily, and the time that remains to breathe out, that is, to exhale air, completely decreases.

Some of the symptoms of obstructive lung diseases are listed below:

a. Wheezing sound
b. Cough

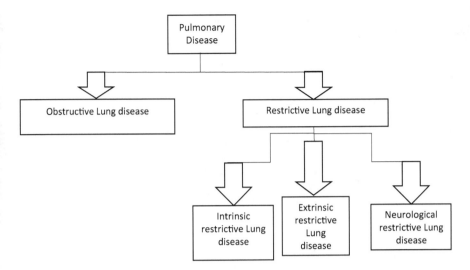

FIGURE 10.1 Types of pulmonary diseases.

   c. Shortness of breath
   d. Increased mucus production
   e. Anxiety

10.2.2 RESTRICTIVE LUNG DISEASE

Restrictive lung disease occurs when the tissue of the chest walls gets damaged, and some other reasons are weakening of muscles, damaged nerves, and so on which restrict the lungs from fully expanding while inhaling gases. Due to restrictive lung disease, there is a huge decrease in a person's ability to inhale air [6]. This can also generate lung stiffness conditions which may worsen a patient's health. Restrictive lung diseases are further classified into three types:

   a. Intrinsic Restrictive Lung disease
   b. Extrinsic Restrictive Lung disease
   c. Neurological Restrictive Lung disease

Intrinsic Restrictive Lung Disease – The disease which occurs due to stiffness in the lungs, and that thus causes a restriction in the functioning of the lungs is called intrinsic restrictive lung disease. For example: pneumonia, tuberculosis and so on.

Extrinsic Restrictive Lung Disease – When the disorder originates from outside of the lungs, then these are termed extrinsic restrictive lung diseases. For example: malignant tumours, obesity, pleurisy and so on.

Neurological Restrictive Lung Disease – This is a disorder in the central nervous system which starts interfering with the air movement of the lungs, and then causes neurological restrictive lung disease. Examples include: muscular dystrophy and paralysis of the diaphragm.

A few prominent symptoms of restrictive lung diseases are listed below:

a. Shortness of breath
b. Cough
c. Anxiety
d. Symptoms of depression

10.3   DIAGNOSIS OF DISEASE AND DISORDER

Most of the symptoms of both restrictive and obstructive diseases overlap with each other. Therefore, the overlap poses one of the most important challenges, which is to differentiate between these two diseases during the process of diagnosis. Machine learning can be beneficial for such a purpose and can show very good results in differentiating in both cases.

Diagnosis is one of the most important factors for the treatment of any disease. An early diagnosis can lead to better results in treatment, as any disease when diagnosed early can be treated better and faster in such a way that it will be less painful for the patient. In some research, it has been found that early detection of diseases can have a high impact on the mortality rate. The earlier the detection, the lower the mortality rate. However, there are a few diseases which cannot be cured completely earlier, and detection provides a very important way to reduce or reverse their effect so that the patient's health can be controlled from getting degraded [7]. Normal clinical procedures sometimes take a long time for diagnosis of a disease as the patient needs to undergo several tests for confirmation.

In the case of pulmonary disorders, there are many traditional clinical methods available for diagnosing the diseases depending upon the condition of the patient. While performing the diagnosis, a few things such as the patient's medical history, symptoms, family medical history, and other physiological signs such as pain are important factors. The patients should also be asked about their daily routine and other matters such as their exposure to gases or their smoking habits.

There are several tests available for the doctor to order, but based on the patient's medical condition, the doctor will advise the required tests one has to undergo. A few tests of the tests used in diagnosing most pulmonary disorders are:

a. Chest X-ray
b. CT Scan
c. SpO2 Level (blood oxygen level)
d. Arterial blood gas analysis
e. Laboratory tests
f. Bronchoscopy
g. Pulmonary function test
h. Sputum test

Among all the tests mentioned above, the one which is mostly used for the diagnosis of pulmonary disorders is the pulmonary function test. Let us discuss all the tests briefly and their applications.

10.4 CHEST X-RAY

The penetration of high energy electromagnetic radiation produces X-radiation. The wavelength of X-rays is shorter than ultra-violet rays, which ranges from 10 picometers to 10 nanometres. To produce X-ray images of the chest, a very low dose of ionizing radiation is used. Patients who are suffering from symptoms like shortness of breath, high fever, injury, cough or pain in the chest are suggested by doctors to have a chest X-ray for diagnosis.

A chest X-ray is used to assess the condition of the chest walls, lungs, heart, bones of chest and spine, blood vessels and airways. It is a non-invasive technique that helps both physicians and doctors as well to diagnose the diseases correctly without causing any pain or discomfort to the patient. Minimal or no special preparation is required to perform a chest X-ray. The chest X-ray will include two views of the patient: one view from the back and the other is supposed to be against the X-ray film. The physiologist will ask the patient to put their hands on their hips, and the chest should be pressed outside against the X-ray plate. If the person is not able to stand, then they should lie down on a table for their chest X-ray to be captured. There are several benefits of X-ray over other techniques, as follows:

a. It is a very fast and easy technique, and hence widely used in cases of emergency.
b. It is a painless method of diagnosis.
c. This method has no side effects.
d. This method is non-invasive.
e. As the machine is inexpensive, this method is affordable.

X-rays are passed carefully over the body to comprehend every small part of an area. The radiation of X-rays is like radio waves, and the number of X-rays absorbed is different for different parts of the body [8]. Bones absorb much of the radiation, while other parts such as soft tissues, fat, muscles and other organs absorb less of X-rays. Therefore, the bones appear white on X-rays, whereas soft tissues appear in shades of grey and air in black colour.

Once an X-ray is done, the physiologist will generate a report and based on the report, doctors will examine the patient and can make the correct diagnosis. A chest X-ray is used for the diagnosis of pulmonary disorders. Some of the diseases which can be diagnosed using chest X-rays are:

a. Lung cancer
b. Pneumonia
c. Fluid collection around lungs
d. Emphysema
e. Air collection around lungs
f. Heart failure

Thus, the X-ray technique can be one of the most important tools for diagnosing pulmonary disorders as it causes minimal discomfort to the patient and is a cost-effective method. In a few cases, the results may not be very useful as only two views

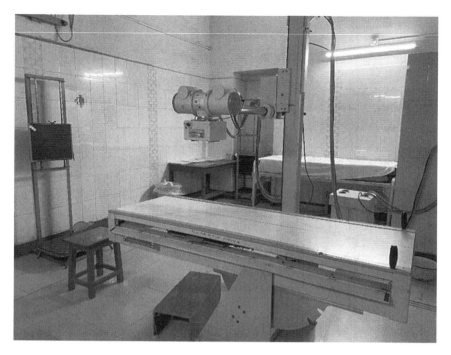

FIGURE 10.2   X-ray machine.

of the chest are used. Figure 10.2 shows a general layout of the X-ray machine. X-ray machines mainly consist of a high-voltage power supply, an X-ray tube and a control console. X-rays are generated by radioisotopes, an X-ray tube and an image detection system, which is comprised of a film and digital capture system. An X-ray tube is a vacuum tube consisting of both an anode and cathode. The cathode is responsible for directing a beam of light into the vacuum. The anode is made up of tungsten, which collects all the electrons to remove heat that is generated by collisions. The radiologist uses a control console to select suitable attributes such as X-ray tube current, voltage, line compensation, exposure time and so on for examining the patient. The image is later produced on an X-ray film. When the patient stands in front of the machine, the rays are passed by an operator. The signal is sent to the signal processing unit, which processes the incoming signal and produces an image on the film. Patients who have a problem with standing or are not well, are allowed to lie down on another machine. This machine follows the same principle as others. The black, grey or white image on the X-ray film primarily depends on two types of X-ray photons, those which pass through the patient without interaction and those which interact.

10.5   CT SCAN

The term CT stands for computerized tomography, which is an advanced form of X-ray technique. X-ray imaging is done from two sides, but in the CT scan, multiple images are taken of the body parts, which are later combined using computers to get a better interpretation of the results. Here, the apparatus uses a rotating X-ray machine to get a cross-sectional image.

The abnormalities which are found in X-rays can be investigated in a more detailed way by using a CT scan. A chest CT scan is used to evaluate injuries and different abnormalities that are found in the chest. In the case of tumours, a CT scan is very important as it will detect to what extent the tumour has spread and also it will evaluate how the tumour is responding to treatment, and accordingly, the radiologist will plan the next session of therapy. Some of the benefits of using a CT scan are:

a. It is a non-invasive technique.
b. It gives accurate results.
c. Use of a CT scan may eliminate the need for biopsy tests and exploratory surgery.
d. It causes no pain to the patient.
e. It is a widely used method for diagnosis.
f. It can get multi-imaging; therefore, it can access bone, soft tissue and blood vessels at a single time.
g. This is a very cost-effective technique.
h. It causes no harm as there is no radiation left inside the patient's body once the examination is done.
i. Unlike X-rays, it is very fast, and therefore helpful for the patient who has a problem holding their breath.
j. It has very little sensitivity concerning the patient's movement.

While a CT scan is being performed, the patient is advised to wear a loose-fitting gown, which is mostly provided by the radiology staff, and for safety purposes, patients are asked to remove all objects which contain metal from their body and to avoid drinking or eating anything a few hours before the test. If required, patients will be injected with a contrast material for which they have to provide all their medical history to the physician. Once the patient is ready, they are asked to lie down on a long examination table which moves in and out of a small tunnel that contains X-ray tubes and electronic X-ray detectors.

The computer is placed in a different room from where the technician is monitoring the scanners. After the completion of the examination, the technician hands over the results to the radiologist, who prepares a report of the diagnosis. This can save patients from undergoing different procedures for the diagnosis of a disease that exhibits different types of symptoms. Thus, a CT scan can be quite useful for the diagnosis of disease as compared to a simple X-ray or any other invasive techniques [9]. The pulmonary diseases which can be diagnosed using a CT scan are:

a. Pneumonia
b. Congenital abnormalities
c. Tuberculosis
d. Benign tumours
e. Malignant tumours

f. Cystic fibrosis
g. Inflammation in the lungs
h. Chronic lung diseases
i. Bronchiectasis
j. Other diseases such as interstitial lung disease, pleura and so on

Thus, a CT scan is a very effective technique for diagnosing various pulmonary diseases as it causes negligible pain to patients while undergoing the procedure. The only concern relevant to the CT scan is sometimes the chance of missing some important data during the multiple imaging and slicing process. In such cases, for confirmation, the doctor may suggest the patient undergo few more tests. To avoid undergoing other tests, machine learning techniques can be used to obtain more accurate results.

Figure 10.3 shows a CT scanning machine. A CT scanner is made up of a gantry, computer and operating console. The gantry consists of all the equipment required for patients and mechanical support. It is made up of X-ray tubes and detectors. Computers are used to collect and analyse data from the detector. The operating console is the master control centre of the CT scanner. The upper layer of the circular region, that is, above the scanner, has detectors that are filled up with gases like xenon and then sealed at both ends. The conductors, which act as a capacitor on the sides, are exposed to high voltage DC. The xenon in the chamber is ionized and then it migrates to the capacitor plate, which causes the current in high voltage load. The current produced is proportional to the radiation and is then fed to the computer for computing images. The CAT scanners take 180 readings at each degree of rotation around a semicircle.

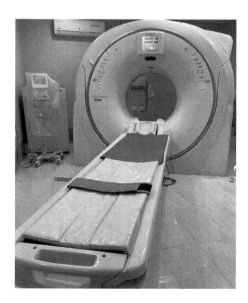

FIGURE 10.3   Computer tomography machine.

10.6 S$_p$O$_2$ LEVEL

The SpO2 level measures the oxygen saturation level in the body, which can be determined using a pulse oximeter, which is a small device that measures the percentage of oxygen in the blood. The reading indicated in a pulse oximeter shows the SpO2 level in the body. The chances of error in the reading of a pulse oximeter is plus or minus two percentages. The doctor may suggest checking the patient's oxygen saturation level if the patient shows the following symptoms:

a. Shortness of breath.
b. If the patient feels extra exertion or a need for extra oxygen while doing a workout.
c. If the patient has breathing difficulties while sleeping.
d. If the patient is suffering from any cardiac problem.

For measuring blood saturation levels, a physician needs a pulse oximeter. This device is very easily available at any medical instrument shop [10]. This device works by sending infrared rays into the capillaries of the inserted part, which may be the finger, toe or earlobe, and is based on the amount of light refracted back off the gases. In this way it measures the blood saturation level in the body. Some of the benefits of using the pulse oximeter device are:

a. It is a portable device, so you can use it anywhere which will help in continuous monitoring of blood oxygen levels.
b. It is cost-effective.
c. It gives a fast result; hence, doctors prefer it.
d. It is used during surgeries for monitoring the oxygen level of patients.

A pulse oximeter is a very small device which can be inserted onto the earlobe, finger or toe. Mostly it is applied on the finger, as that is the most convenient area for measurement. If the patient is wearing any nail polish, then the technician will ask to remove it. An examination done over dark nail polish or in extremely cold weather conditions will show a SpO2 level lower than normal. This device is very useful for the primary indication and identification of causes of symptoms. Diseases which can be indicated by using a pulse oximeter are:

a. Chronic obstructive pulmonary disease
b. Covid-19
c. Asthma
d. Pneumonia
e. Heart failure
f. Sleep apnea

This test will only give the patient a prior indication that there are chances of some abnormalities in the functioning of your lungs, based on which your doctor will suggest you undergo a series of tests that can be time-consuming. The use of machine learning techniques can be a time saver in such cases.

10.7   ARTERIAL BLOOD GAS ANALYSIS

The amount of oxygen carried out by our red blood cells can be measured by calculating the blood oxygen level. For maintaining good health, it is very important to have a good oxygen level. The body itself functions in a way to maintain a good oxygen level. If the oxygen level and the amount of gases in the body do not remain at the appropriate level, then this will affect the functioning of the body, which can further cause various symptoms and indicate some health problems mainly related to the pulmonary system or in some cases also the cardiac system.

For the simple measurement of the blood saturation level, the pulse oximeter can be used to calculate the oxygen level, but if the physician wants to see the number of other gases inside the body and how their values vary, it is not possible to use a pulse oximeter for this purpose as it can only tell about the oxygen level. Hence, arterial blood gas (ABG) analysis is another test that is used to measure the different levels of gases inside the body. Arterial blood gas analysis is a laboratory test, and in this test, blood is drawn from the artery. The arterial blood gas analysis also measures the amount of acid and base level in the body, which helps to calculate pH level [11]. The doctor will advise the patients to have an arterial blood gas analysis done if the following symptoms are seen:

a. Chest pain
b. Rapid heartbeat
c. Confusion
d. Headache

In arterial blood gas analysis, blood is not drawn from veins because the veins do not contain oxygenated blood. Also, in the arteries, unlike the veins, one can feel the pulse. The arteries in the wrist are used for collecting a sample of arterial blood gas of the patient. A few diseases which can be indicated using the results of this test are:

a. Pulmonary embolism
b. Acute respiratory distress syndrome
c. Anaemia
d. Cyanosis
e. Heart diseases
f. Emphysema

Patients with a history of smoking generally show a high pulse due to the deposition of carbon monoxide in the body. For such patients, it is necessary to have arterial blood gas analysis as a pulse oximeter cannot detect differences in other gases. The normal reading for arterial blood gas analysis of healthy patients should lie between 80 and 100 millimetres of mercury (mm Hg).

10.8   LABORATORY TESTS

Some of the most common laboratory tests are a complete blood count (CBC) and a comprehensive metabolic panel. These tests help evaluate blood cells and also tell how well your body organs are functioning. After assessing the results of a CBC, arterial blood gas (ABG), and comprehensive metabolic panel (CMP) tests a lung condition may be suspected, and depending on the results, the doctor may suggest you to undergo some specialized tests for the proper diagnosis of causes.

A cystic fibrosis test is suggested by the doctor to check whether the amount of chloride in sweat should be tested in the patient. For diagnosis purposes, a cystic fibrosis sweat test is the standard test and an Alpha-1 antitrypsin is a test that measures the deficiency of Alpha-1 antitrypsin in the body, which another cause of chronic obstructive pulmonary disease (COPD). In cases where there is a build-up of extra fluid around the lung and chest wall, a pleural fluid analysis test is used to diagnose whether it is cancer or infection. In this test, a sample of fluid is collected which will be later tested for a final diagnosis. For determining triggers of asthma, an allergy test is used. A few other tests will also be suggested by the doctor for the diagnosis of causes of infections and some of them are:

a. Targeted testing for a virus
b. Targeted testing for bacteria
c. Targeted testing for fungi
d. Serologic testing
e. Respiratory pathogen panels
f. Culture tests

Several other important tests are based on auto antibody tests if the patient is suffering from an autoimmune disorder that affects the lungs. In case of the need to evaluate cancer, a lung tissue biopsy test is done in which a small sample of tissue is used for assessing lung condition. Again, to test that a patient is suffering from which type of antibody disorder, a few more tests may be advised [12]. In such cases, machine learning can be beneficial as the methods will help to obtain faster results.

10.9 BRONCHOSCOPY

Bronchi are the main pathways of the lungs, and doctors advise bronchoscopy to examine the inside of the lungs. This procedure helps the doctor to examine the pathways of the lungs. Bronchoscopy is a procedure which the patient undergoes and recovers quickly from. This procedure requires a few preparations, and the patient may be recommended to have bronchoscopy due to the following reasons:

a. Coughing up blood
b. Blockage in airways
c. For transplant purposes
d. Chronic cough
e. Examination of tumour
f. Need of biopsy

During bronchoscopy, the doctor first uses a spray to the throat and nasal area to numb that area, so the patient will not feel any pain. Once the area gets numb, the doctor insert a flexible tube into the throat and nose [13]. The patient will feel like coughing as the tube starts to move inside. As a precaution, doctors also have oxygen available to them during the procedure. In cases where the doctor needs to take a biopsy, bronchoscopy is used. In a biopsy, a small piece of tissue is taken from the affected area to examine it further. For a biopsy, the doctor may insert a needle and brush, along with another required instrument, which will be inserted inside the nose and throat using a channel in the bronchoscope.

Lights and cameras are also attached to see clearly around the bends. The doctor may also take an ultrasound during this procedure to have a clear picture of tissues and lymph nodes around the bronchi. To examine cells and fluid, the doctor sprays a saline solution during a process called bronchial lavage. Diseases which can be diagnosed after this procedure are:

a. Cancer
b. Viral infection
c. Fungi
d. Lung damage
e. Bacterial infection
f. Narrowing of bronchi
g. Narrowing of trachea

This procedure is mostly suggested to a patient after the results of an X-ray or CT scan are obtained. If some abnormalities are found in the results of these scans, then the doctor may suggest the patient undergo this bronchoscopy procedure. This is an invasive technique and patients may feel discomfort during this procedure, and some may also develop side effects like breathing difficulties, infection, fever, minor bleeding and so on. In such cases, machine learning techniques can give results in a few steps with more accuracy as it gives results based on detected patterns. Thus, using such procedures can be avoided and a confirmatory test is mainly used for any disease. Use of machine learning can help the patient to get a diagnosis much earlier.

10.10   SPUTUM TEST

The windpipe splits into different channels called bronchi, and it starts at the back of the throat and is connected to the lungs. The body produces sputum if the area between the lungs and the mouth gets irritated due to any reason [14]. Sputum is also called phlegm. The growth of substances like fungi and bacteria generates sputum. The production and accumulation of saliva make breathing difficult and can also cause a cough. The doctor may suggest that the patient undergo a sputum test if they show the following symptoms:

a. Muscle aches
b. Chest pain
c. Cough
d. Fever
e. Confusion

f. Fatigue
g. Breathing difficulties
h. Chills

A bit of preparation is required before giving a sample for the sputum test. The doctor will advise the patient to skip a meal before giving sputum. The patient is also advised to rinse their mouth properly before sample collection. The doctor will also check if the patient is on any medication which contains bacteria-killing antibiotics or not. If yes, then the doctor will ask them to skip a dose before the test. The pathologist will provide the patient with a clean cup and ask them to cough up some sputum into it. If the patient is not able to do so by themselves, then doctor will collect the sample by using a bronchoscope. Once the sample is collected, doctor will try to analyse its colour. Green, off-white and yellow colours indicate lung infections. Black and grey colours indicate exposure to smoke and dust. Similarly, rusty and red colours indicate some serious conditions. Diseases which can be diagnosed by sputum test are:

a. Lung abscess
b. Tuberculosis
c. Cystic fibrosis
d. Bronchitis
e. Pneumonia
f. Chronic obstructive pulmonary disease

The sample needs to be stored very carefully as there is a high chance of contamination. Also, if the patient is on any medication, the prior use of antibiotics can inhibit the growth of abnormalities. The results of this test get delayed sometimes and the use of machine learning techniques can help in the automatic detection of disease by using the dataset.

10.11   PULMONARY FUNCTION TEST

The pulmonary function test is used to assess the capacity of the lungs in human beings. It is also known as spirometry. This test calculates the volume of the lungs, the rate of flow and how the exchange of gases takes place. This test is very useful in diagnosing and differentiating obstructive and restrictive diseases. The doctor will suggest the patient undergo pulmonary function testing (PFT) test (as shown in Figure 10.4) if the following symptoms are seen:

a. History of exposure to smoke
b. Symptoms of a lung problem
c. Monitoring required for the condition of COPD and asthma
d. The need to access lungs before surgery

Doctors will advise the patient to stop taking any medications before undergoing this test, as medicines can cause variations in the actual result. A PFT technician will

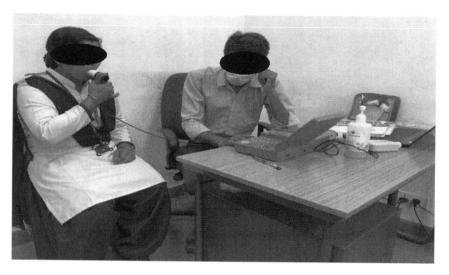

FIGURE 10.4 Pulmonary function test.

ask the patient to sit up straight and keep a mouthpiece between their teeth and close it with their mouth. First, the patient inhales the air infill in the lungs for six seconds and when asked by the technician, exhales air continuously for 10–15 seconds and again inhales quickly [15]. Once this procedure is completed, the technician will give the patient a bronchodilator and ask them to wait for six minutes. After six minutes, the same test is repeated again, and this is called a pre-PFT and post-PFT test. This test is done twice to see the effect in the functioning of the lungs after the broncho-dilator. This test measures:

a. FEV1 – Amount of air exhaled in first second
b. FVC – Total amount of air exhaled forcefully
c. FEV1/FVC – Ratio of the amount of air exhaled in the first second to the total air exhale
d. FEF – Average rate of flow
e. PEF – The highest rate at which patient can force out air from their lungs
f. TLC – Total lung capacity
g. VC – Vital capacity, which measures the total air the patient can exhale after inhaling
h. FRC – Functional residual capacity, that is, amounts of air left inside the lungs after exhaling normally
i. Residual Volume – The amount of air left after exhaling forcefully

The pulmonary function test is a non-invasive technique and causes no pain to the patient. Diseases which can be identified using pulmonary function tests are:

a. Asthma
b. Chronic obstructive pulmonary disease

c. Bronchiectasis
d. Asbestosis
e. Lung fibrosis
f. Allergies
g. Chronic bronchitis
h. Sarcoidosis
i. Respiratory infection
j. The weakening of chest wall muscles

The boundaries in differentiating diseases using PFT results is very thin, so there are chances that sometimes a disease might not be diagnosed correctly. Applying machine learning techniques and using computerized analysis, we can get automatic and correct interpretation of diseases in a very short amount of time.

10.12   CHALLENGES AND ISSUES

One of the biggest challenges in the field of medicine is early diagnosis. How well a patient will respond to treatment majorly depends upon how early they have been diagnosed with a disease. Sometimes, for example, a lung cancer patient may not show major symptoms until the final stage, but observing those small daily life symptoms and difficulties and going directly for a test which gives a clear diagnosis is something our medical systems are still lagging in. This trial-and-error method of diagnosing diseases by trying numerous tests sometimes becomes very tedious for a patient who is already not fit physically.

Let us take the examples of asthma and COPD, both of which show almost the same symptoms. If the reports of a PFT show reversibility, then the patient will get a clear diagnosis. Reversibility might not be clearly visible in many cases, however, due to issues such as the patient having already used an inhaler, there being an error by a technician, or the patient may not have performed well [16]. In such cases, the application of machine learning techniques can provide much better results. Asthma and COPD can be differentiated minutely with the help of patient medical history, the patient's family history, if they are exposed to smoke or not, allergies and so on. Also, lung sounds can also help in diagnosing the disease [17]. If the machine learning technique is used to develop a computerized model which when trained with such a large number of dataset and parameters can give a diagnosis, then it will be very much helpful for both doctors and patients.

Similarly, in the case of a CT scan, if the programme is designed and the system is trained through a machine learning technique to analyse images of scans using a database, then it can provide better and much faster results. Also, a training system using a dataset of CT scans along with ultrasounds can be very beneficial as the system will give an accurate result [18]. Such an application of machine learning techniques can also eliminate the use of invasive techniques which at times can be painful and uncomfortable for patients. Using machine learning techniques will also eliminate the chances of human error while performing any test or preparation of reports [19].

10.13   APPLICATION OF MACHINE LEARNING IN DIAGNOSIS OF PULMONARY DISORDER

Machine learning techniques have been considered as most useful techniques in recent years. Machine learning algorithms have shown effective results in various applications [20]. In cases of pulmonary disorders, machine learning techniques can be useful for the diagnosis of diseases employing two major techniques:

    a. Image processing
    b. Signal processing

In patient care, both in terms of diagnosis and treatment, radiologic imaging is increasing rapidly. Intelligent and automated image analysis are becoming very important for real radiologic practices which involve segmentation, registration, computer-aided diagnosis (CAD), and detection. Treatment and diagnosis can be improved by using imaging technology. The CT scan, magnetic resonance imagining (MRI), X-ray, ultrasound and so on are some of the widely used techniques in radiological scanning centres. Based on the applications, machine learning techniques can be classified as supervised, unsupervised and semi-supervised learning [21]. The machine learning technique has various models that can be used for diagnosis. Linear models, learning with kernels, the probabilistic model, dimensionality reduction and cluster analysis are some of the models of machine learning. Figure 10.5 depicts the steps of using image processing through employing machine learning in the diagnosis of disease.

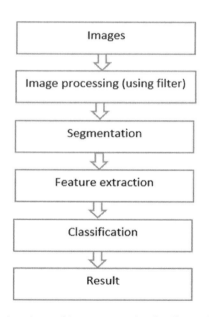

FIGURE 10.5   Machine learning and image processing for diagnosis result of disorder.

For classification purposes, there are several techniques which are available as machine learning methods such as support vector machine (SVM), naive Bayes classifiers, decision tree, logistic regression and etc. Some of the features which can be extracted using imaging techniques are entropy, picture to signal noise ratio (PSNR), correlation, homogeneity and so on [22]. Lung auscultation has been the oldest method for the detection of pulmonary disorders. Patient respiratory function can be identified by using lung auscultation [23]. There are chances of error in diagnosis when hearing lung sounds in real time due to several factors like surroundings in the clinic, patient's ability to inhale-exhale and so on. Emerging technologies can lead to the development of a powerful computerized-based respiratory sound analysis system to diagnose abnormalities in respiratory sounds [24]. For computerized-based respiratory sound analysis, an electronic stethoscope is required to record auscultations in real time.

Figure 10.6 shows various steps involved in the classification of a disorder using signal processing methods that employ machine learning techniques. The captured data which is medical imaging modality, is subjected to some pre-processing methods for making the images suitable for further stages. Then, the feature extraction is done, and the appropriate features are selected. These features are utilized in the classification application, which helps in the diagnosis process of the analysis of disorder. The computerized-based respiratory sound analysis encompasses different machine learning techniques like neural network, classifier ensemble methods, decision trees, and support vector machine [25, 26]. Some of the important features which can be extracted from lung sounds are standard deviation, mean, RMS value, skewness, kurtosis, crest factor, maximum frequency, dominant frequency, formant frequency,

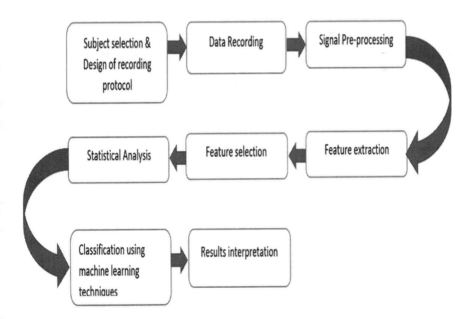

FIGURE 10.6   Signal processing using machine learning.

spectral centroid and so on. Machine learning tools have been effective tools for researchers in past years for the diagnosis of diseases. The use of machine learning techniques will support medical professionals in diagnosing patients efficiently. Machine learning methods assist in improved diagnosis performance and efficient CAD implementation for medical image analysis, processing and diagnosis [27].

10.14   CONCLUSION

This chapter discusses the background, cause and impact of pulmonary disorder, which is a major cause of lung cancers across the world. The different scanning and test techniques have also been discussed. Finally, the role of machine learning used along with signal processing and image processing techniques have been discussed.

LEARNING OUTCOMES

At the end of studying this chapter, students and learners will be able to:

- Explain the background and cause of lung cancer
- Elaborate tests and scanning methods for pulmonary disorder
- Highlight issues and challenges in conventional methods of diagnosis
- Interpret the role of machine learning with signal processing for improved diagnosis results

EXERCISE FOR PRACTICE AND DISCUSSION

1. Enumerate the traditional methods of diagnosis and screening of lung cancers. Also discuss the major shortcoming in these conventional diagnosis methods for addressing the issues of pulmonary disorder.
2. Early detection of disorders can save many lives; thus, explain how machine learning can play a significant role in achieving early detection.
3. Feature extraction methods are used to obtain appropriate sets of features used in the classification of disease, but only selected features are useful in the classification. Explain.
4. What are the major challenges and issues in various types of tests and screening methods used in analysis of pulmonary disorder?

REFERENCES

1. Nakahira, K., Pabon Porras, M. A., & Choi, A. M. (2016). Autophagy in pulmonary diseases. *American Journal of Respiratory and Critical Care Medicine, 194*(10), 1196–1207.
2. James, A. L., & Wenzel, S. (2007). Clinical relevance of airway remodelling in airway diseases. *European Respiratory Journal, 30*(1), 134–155.
3. Castelino, F. V., & Varga, J. (2010). Interstitial lung disease in connective tissue diseases: Evolving concepts of pathogenesis and management. *Arthritis Research & Therapy, 12*(4), 213. https://doi.org/10.1186/ar3097

4. Aviado, D. M. (2013). *The lung circulation: Pathologic physiology and therapy of diseases.* Elsevier.
5. Chabat, F., Yang, G. Z., & Hansell, D. M. (2003). Obstructive lung diseases: Texture classification for differentiation at CT. *Radiology, 228*(3), 871–877.
6. Mannino, D. M., Ford, E. S., & Redd, S. C. (2003). Obstructive and restrictive lung disease and markers of inflammation: Data from the Third National Health and Nutrition Examination. *The American Journal of Medicine, 114*(9), 758–762.
7. Stout, J. E., Koh, W. J., & Yew, W. W. (2016). Update on pulmonary disease due to nontuberculous mycobacteria. *International Journal of Infectious Diseases, 45*, 123–134.
8. Swingler, G. H., Du Toit, G., Andronikou, S., Van der Merwe, L., & Zar, H. J. (2005). Diagnostic accuracy of chest radiography in detecting mediastinal lymphadenopathy in suspected pulmonary tuberculosis. *Archives of Disease in Childhood, 90*(11), 1153–1156.
9. Blanchon, T., Bréchot, J. M., Grenier, P. A., Ferretti, G. R., Lemarié, E., Milleron, B., ... & Blanchon, F. (2007). Baseline results of the Depiscan study: A French randomized pilot trial of lung cancer screening comparing low dose CT scan (LDCT) and chest X-ray (CXR). *Lung Cancer, 58*(1), 50–58.
10. Banks, M. R., Kumar, P. J., & Mulcahy, H. E. (2001). Pulse oximetry saturation levels during routine unsedated diagnostic upper gastrointestinal endoscopy. *Scandinavian Journal of Gastroenterology, 36*(1), 105–109.
11. Stein, P. D., Goldhaber, S. Z., Henry, J. W., & Miller, A. C. (1996). Arterial blood gas analysis in the assessment of suspected acute pulmonary embolism. *Chest, 109*(1), 78–81.
12. Hampson, N. B. (1995, September). Pulmonary embolism: Difficulties in the clinical diagnosis. *Seminars in Respiratory Infections, 10*(3), 123–130.
13. Prakash, U. B., & Matthay, R. A. (1994). Bronchoscopy. *Journal of Bronchology & Interventional Pulmonology, 1*(4), 340–349.
14. Albert, H., Heydenrych, A., Brookes, R., Mole R J., Harley, B., Subotsky, E., ... & Azevedo, V. (2002). Performance of a rapid phage-based test, FASTPlaqueTB™, to diagnose pulmonary tuberculosis from sputum specimens in South Africa. *The International Journal of Tuberculosis and Lung Disease, 6*(6), 529–537.
15. Singh, D., Singh, B. K., & Behera, A. K. (2020, January). Comparative analysis of Lung sound denoising technique. In IEEE (Ed.), *2020 First International Conference on Power, Control and Computing Technologies (ICPC2T)* (pp. 406–410). IEEE.
16. Culver, B. H., Graham, B. L., Coates, A. L., Wanger, J., Berry, C. E., Clarke, P. K., ... & McCormack, M. C. (2017). Recommendations for a standardized pulmonary function report. An official American Thoracic Society technical statement. *American Journal of Respiratory and Critical Care Medicine, 196*(11), 1463–1472.
17. Gurung, A., Scrafford, C. G., Tielsch, J. M., Levine, O. S., & Checkley, W. (2011). Computerized lung sound analysis as diagnostic aid for the detection of abnormal lung sounds: A systematic review and meta-analysis. *Respiratory Medicine, 105*(9), 1396–1403.
18. Menon, U., Gentry-Maharaj, A., Hallett, R., Ryan, A., Burnell, M., Sharma, A., ... & Godfrey, K. (2009). Sensitivity and specificity of multimodal and ultrasound screening for ovarian cancer, and stage distribution of detected cancers: results of the prevalence screen of the UK Collaborative Trial of Ovarian Cancer Screening (UKCTOCS). *The Lancet Oncology, 10*(4), 327–340.
19. Fatima, M., & Pasha, M. (2017). Survey of machine learning algorithms for disease diagnostic. *Journal of Intelligent Learning Systems and Applications, 9*(1), 1–16.

20. Wang, S., & Summers, R. M. (2012). Machine learning and radiology. *Medical Image Analysis, 16*(5), 933–951.

21. Makaju, S., Prasad, P. W. C., Alsadoon, A., Singh, A. K., & Elchouemi, A. (2018). Lung cancer detection using CT scan images. *Procedia Computer Science, 125,* 107–114.

22. Kim, S. Y., Diggans, J., Pankratz, D., Huang, J., Pagan, M., Sindy, N., ... & Steele, M. P. (2015). Classification of usual interstitial pneumonia in patients with interstitial lung disease: assessment of a machine learning approach using high-dimensional transcriptional data. *The Lancet Respiratory Medicine, 3*(6), 473–482.

23. Palaniappan, R., Sundaraj, K., & Ahamed, N. U. (2013). Machine learning in lung sound analysis: a systematic review. *Biocybernetics and Biomedical Engineering, 33*(3), 129–135.

24. Palaniappan, R., Sundaraj, K., Ahamed, N. U., Arjunan, A., & Sundaraj, S. (2013). Computer-based respiratory sound analysis: a systematic review. *IETE Technical Review, 30*(3), 248–256.

25. İçer, S., & Gengeç, Ş. (2014). Classification and analysis of non-stationary characteristics of crackle and rhonchus lung adventitious sounds. *Digital Signal Processing, 28,* 18–27.

26. Haider, N. S., Singh, B. K., Periyasamy, R., & Behera, A. K. (2019). Respiratory sound based classification of chronic obstructive pulmonary disease: A risk stratification approach in machine learning paradigm. *Journal of Medical Systems, 43,* 255. https://doi.org/10.1007/s10916-019-1388-0

27. Sinha, G. R., & Patel, Bhagwati (2014). *Medical image processing: Concepts and applications.* Prentice Hall of India.

11 Mental Illness and Neurodevelopmental Disorders

LEARNING OBJECTIVES

The chapter aims to:

- Present an overview of various neurodevelopmental disorders
- Discuss developmental dyslexia and diagnostic methods
- Understand attention-deficit/hyperactivity disorder (ADHD)
- Elaborate Parkinson's disease, epilepsy and schizophrenia

11.1 NEURODEVELOPMENTAL DISORDERS

Neurodevelopmental disorders are associated to any abnormality in the function of the brain during its growing phases [1]. At times, children's brain tends to change, modify and establish connections in its developmental stages based on the information it gathers from the developing environment. So, a complete understanding of the developing brain in its development stages is necessary, to understand any abnormal function at the early stage. Children with disorders often develop difficulty in learning, emotion processing, hearing and vision. Examples of neurodevelopmental disorders are attention deficit/hyperactivity disorder (ADHD), autism spectrum disorder (ASD), learning disability (LD), intellectual disability, cerebral palsy and impairment in vision and hearing. Among all of these, ADHD, ASD and LD are the most common developmental disorders. An appropriate treatment can help provide a complete cure for some developmental disorders, whereas others are persistent and essential therapy can possibly reduce the symptoms to an extent.

11.2 DEVELOPMENTAL DYSLEXIA

Developmental dyslexia (DD) is one of the neurodevelopmental disorders which affect the reading skills in children despite a normal IQ [1]. Dyslexia is considered to be the most common learning disability found in children and adults. Developmental dyslexia often refers to reduced phonological processing deficit and is interrelated with complexity in processing the sound structure (phonology) with the written word form, which causes a deficit in developing reading activities in dyslexic children.

DOI: 10.1201/9781003097808-11

There is a lack of continual progress in tasks related to reading and learning in schoolchildren, and this makes it difficult for them to mix with other children who are normal, leading to psychological issues at early ages. So early detection of dyslexia may stop dyslexic children from experiencing social and psychological issues and enhance their personality and academic performance. Some common dyslexia symptoms are:

- Delay in talking
- Poor reading and writing skills
- Reversal of letters
- Slow learning
- Poor handwriting (difficult to read)
- Spelling mistakes
- Poor academic performance

Reading is a complex cognitive process that requires different skills such as visual, attention and linguistic processing, and interaction from different brain areas. The reading circuitry of the brain is composed of several neural systems which support language as well as the word recognition and visual process, attention, working memory, comprehension, motor functions and cognition [1]. Like most brain disorders, dyslexia causes abnormalities in functions or structures in some brain areas. The discovery of abnormally functioning areas of dyslexic brains would enable researchers to focus their study on those areas. Several neuroimaging methods such as functional magnetic resonance imaging (fMRI), magnetoencephalography (MEG), electroencephalography (EEG) and functional near-infrared spectroscopy (fNIRS) have shown the regions which are responsible for reading. Studies have found activation of brain regions lateralized towards the left hemisphere (language areas) in normal readers during reading tasks, and also researchers found the recruitment of the left fusiform gyrus area (visual word form area) in experienced readers which engages during orthographic and phonological processing [2]. These brain areas are referred to as reading circuitry in the brain, which grows as children acquires specific skills in reading, and these and other skills related to reading are found to be compromised in dyslexic individuals [1] [2].

11.2.1 Diagnostic Methods

The diagnostic methods in dyslexia can be broadly categorized into two, namely, behavioural methods and brain imaging methods.

11.2.2 Behavioural Method

The behavioural method is the most common and popular method available presently for the diagnosis of dyslexia. The behavioural method is based on the standardized test battery used by psychologists to assess an individual based on behaviour patterns and symptoms. The test battery assess the individual's skills in decoding, phonological awareness, comprehension, rapid naming and reading fluency. Psychologists make their evaluation based on the scores obtained in the test along with the individual's family history and biographical details. The symptoms may vary from person to person and also the severity varies from mild to severe.

11.2.3 BRAIN IMAGING MODALITIES

In brain imaging methods, psychologists/clinicians use brain imaging modalities like EEG, fMRI, MEG and positron emission tomography (PET) to view the distinct behavioural patterns in brain images/signals. These methods are still in the experimental stage, and many studies have shown distinct anatomical and behavioural patterns in the dyslexic brain compared to typical developing children.

With advancements in technology and machine learning algorithms, researchers in recent times have become interested in identifying and classifying the different anatomical structures and patterns which are unique to dyslexic brain. Researchers use fMRI and diffusion tensor imaging (DTI) images to study the differences in white and grey matter (anatomical structures) in the dyslexic brain compared to the normal brain. Another approach is to analyse the brain signals as in an EEG and MEG in order to study the functional response of the dyslexic brain with respect to given stimuli or during rest. Functional connectivity is one of the methods to study the activation and interactions of different brain areas during tasks and at rest periods.

11.2.4 RECENT ADVANCEMENT IN DIAGNOSTIC TECHNIQUES

With the recent development in computation and machine learning techniques, many researchers are using machine learning techniques to predict and diagnose dyslexia using physiological data. Since many physicians are following manual techniques for diagnosis, machine learning algorithms are expected to help clinicians acquire equal expert knowledge in automated diagnosis of dyslexia. Khan et al. [3] presented an automated classification system for the diagnosis of dyslexia in 857 school children and found 98% accuracy using the K-neighbours classifier in classifying their own datasets into two groups (non-dyslexics and suspicious for dyslexia). Asvestopoulou et al. [4] developed a screening tool for dyslexia detection using eye movements. The authors used an eye tracking method (i.e. tracking aberrant eye movements during reading) for dyslexia detection which is different from the usual detection methods like behavioural and brain imaging methods, and found the best classification performance in a linear SVM model with 97% accuracy in classifying dyslexic children from normal children.

In another study, Tamboer et al. [5] showed the possibility of ML techniques in classifying dyslexic young adults and normal adults using brain anatomical scans. The authors used an SVM classifier for classification and attained 80% classification accuracy on the differences in grey matter. Certain regions were found such as the left inferior parietal lobule, and left and right occipital fusiform gyrus were more reliable in classification and the researchers stated that these regions could be effectively used as biomarkers in dyslexia detection. Pavithran et al. [6] demonstrated the usefulness of the theta/alpha ratio in identifying the visual attention deficit in dyslexia using a task-based EEG. In this study, the authors found a positive correlation between the theta/alpha ratio with the visual deficit in dyslexic children and concluded that an increased theta/alpha ratio is largely associated with impaired visual orientation while identifying two different spatial target stimuli. Recently, Seshadri et al. [7] analysed the nodal activation in dyslexic children using resting EEG data and found increased EEG theta node strength at the temporal, parietal and occipital regions during rest time. In this study, the authors concluded that increased theta node strength during rest could be a biomarker to identify resting state functional impairments in dyslexia. Figure 11.1 shows the steps involved in the detection of dyslexia based on behavioural and neurobiological data.

Although soft computing and machine learning techniques are frequently used in the detection of many clinical disorders, their effectiveness in dyslexia detection is

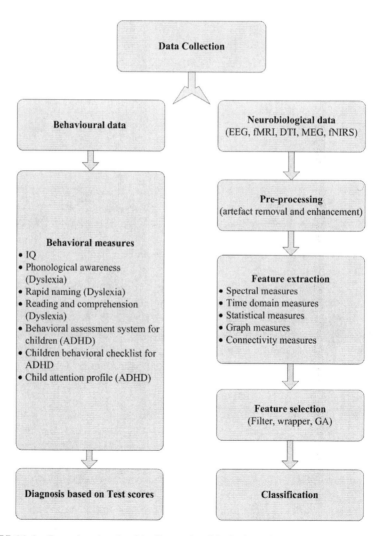

FIGURE 11.1   Procedure involved in diagnosis of dyslexia and ADHD.

yet be studied broadly. Also, as the most emerging machine learning technique, one could use deep learning techniques to classify or detect dyslexia at early ages.

11.3 ATTENTION-DEFICIT/HYPERACTIVITY DISORDER (ADHD)

Attention-deficit/hyperactivity disorder (ADHD) is the most common neurodevelopmental disorder found in children. ADHD is a disorder with impulsive behaviour and hyperactivity, with severe trouble in sustaining attention [8]. It affects more than 5% of children around the globe and it has no cure. ADHD is seen in children and may persist into adulthood if it's not treated. ADHD is more commonly observed in boys than girls. Several researchers around the globe are still exploring the causes for ADHD. However, present research findings argue that interactions among genes and environmental factors have a significant effect on brain development during the prenatal phase [9]. Also, there are non-genetic factors which could be the cause of ADHD. A few common causes for ADHD are listed below:

- Genes
- Smoking
- Consumption of alcohol and drugs during pregnancy
- Exposure to environmental toxins, such as high levels of lead, at a young age
- Low birthweight
- Brain injuries

11.3.1 TYPES

- Mostly impulsive hyperactive
- Mostly inattentive
- Combined

11.3.2 SYMPTOMS

ADHD is diagnosed according to the 18 symptoms defined by the 10th edition of the *International Classification of the Diseases* (ICD-10) [10] and the 5th edition of the *Diagnostic and Statistical Manual of Mental Disorders* [8] to observe inattention, hyperactivity and impulsive behaviours.

Inattention:

- Lack of attention to details and often makes mistakes carelessly in school and other tasks
- Trouble in sustaining attention while playing or doing any work (reduced or lack of focused attention)
- Not attentive and fails to pay attention when speaking to directly
- Easily distracted during tasks and fails to follow given instructions
- Displays poor task and activity management
- Exhibits disinterest and avoid tasks that require constant mental effort
- Fails to remember stuffs related to essential activities

- Easily distracted by irrelevant things/thoughts
- Fails to remember normal everyday activities.

Hyperactivity and impulsivity:

- Frequently taps or fidgets using hands/feet or squirms in seat.
- Does not stay seated in one place; often leaves seat when being seated is required
- Feels restless
- Quite difficult to engage in a task or in leisure activity
- Is often "on the go," acting as if "driven by a motor"
- Talks too much
- Blurts out an answer often even before a question is completed
- Has difficulty in waiting for turn
- Interrupts frequently with others

Based on the symptoms, the clinicians categorize the severity of ADHD into mild, moderate and severe cases. Also, there's a high probability for comorbid condition for ADHD with other disorders like conduct disorder, learning disabilities, anxiety, depression and oppositional defiant disorders.

11.3.3   ADHD Screening

There's no specific test for ADHD, but there are several screening methods, which include behavioural tests, questionnaire and interview-based tests and psychological tests. Some common tests used by psychologists in children [11] are:

- Child Behavioural Checklist for ADHD (CBCL)
- Behavior Assessment System for Children (BASC)
- The Child Attention Profile
- The Vanderbilt Assessment Scale

Some common tests used in adults [11] are:

- Adult ADHD Self-Report Scale (ASRS-v1.1)
- Conners Adult ADHD Rating Scales (CAARS)
- Brown Attention-Deficit Disorder Scale (BADDS) for adults

11.3.4   Diagnosis Based on Brain Imaging and Machine Learning Methods

With the recent progress in neuro-imaging, several researchers have investigated the brain images and signals from ADHD subjects in order to identify the abnormal or distinct functional brain areas compared to individuals without ADHD. Up until now, the diagnosis of ADHD was based on questionnaires and interviews by clinicians, which are more subjective, and therefore the identification of bio/neural markers would largely support clinicians to make a clear decision.

Also, with the recent development in computing methods, researchers have become interested in classifying the differences in the brain regions that are associated to ADHD in children. Dai et al. [12] came up with an automated classification framework for ADHD with the help of MRI image features, and also these authors have studied the effect of different features in classifying ADHD and proposed a multi-modal framework for efficient classification of ADHD. Guven et al. [13] investigated the efficiency of combined EEG-fNIRS in classifying ADHD children. Authors have found the best classification accuracy, of 93.18%, using combined EEG-fNIRS features compared to using EEG features alone with 79.14% accuracy. Iannaccone et al. [14] used multiple discriminative structural and functional brain maps to classify ADHD individuals from controls. The authors used a flanker/Nogo task to analyse inhibition and error processing as functional features. The functional features along with the structural brain data were fed to a support vector machine (SVM) pattern recognition algorithm for classification. In this research, the authors obtained classification accuracy of 77.78% based on functional features and also identified brain regions such as the occipital cortex, temporal cortex and posterior cingulate as better predictive regions for ADHD.

Ariyarathne et al. [15] employed a convolutional neural network (CNN) with a seed-based approach to identify ADHD subjects using resting fMRI data. In this study, the authors proposed a method using seed-correlation analysis to compute functional connectivity between a seed region and all voxel areas. This seed correlation was then used for classification using a CNN and achieved a classification accuracy of 84% to 86% for four major brain regions.

Recently, Moghaddari et al. [16] proposed a method for ADHD diagnosis using CNN with task-based EEG data. The authors recorded EEGs for 30 ADHD children and 31 normal children during mental task performance and converted all the extracted EEG bands to coloured RGB images. The images were then imported to a 13-layer CNN model for extracting features and classifying the groups. In this study, the authors obtained average classification accuracy of 98.48% and found better performance of their model compared to previous results. Figure 11.1 depicts the steps involved in detection of ADHD based on behavioural and neurobiological data. Though neuroimaging research has been widely used in studying different research works in the area of identification of ADHD, it is still in the experimental stage and the results have not been validated with conclusive research evidence in diagnosing ADHD.

11.3.5 Treatment for ADHD

Behavioural therapy and medication are the major treatment methods for treating ADHD. Psychologists and trained professionals in special schools provide behavioural therapy to children and parents to aid them in monitoring and improving the behaviour of the children. Medication such as stimulants and non-stimulants are used to treat ADHD and have shown better results by controlling nervous system responses. These medications are normally recommended by doctors have many benefits with some side effects also. Some common medications used to treat ADHD are methylphenidate (Ritalin), amphetamine-based stimulants (Adderall), atomoxetine (Strattera), and some antidepressants such as bupropion (Wellbutrin).

11.4 PARKINSON'S DISEASE

Parkinson's disease (PD) is a neurodegenerative disorder which mainly affects the neuro-motor area of the brain. Parkinson's disease is the second most common disorder after Alzheimer's disease among elderly people (usually over the age of 55 years). The patient suffering from PD may face problems in controlling the movement, balancing and maintaining body posture. It is termed a disorder of weakness and tremors [17]. The disease is named after a British doctor, James Parkinson, who first described it in the year 1817. If we look at the epidemiology of PD, the prevalence rate is 0.5–1% in the age group 65–69 years, which further increases to 1–3% in persons age 80 years and older [18], [19]. A study in this field has predicted the number of PD cases will double by the year 2030 [20].

The most common motor symptom of PD is bradykinesia, which is slow movement of muscles. This is the result of the insufficient signalling of dopamine due to the degeneration process of neurons that generate the dopamine compound in the substantia-nigra region of the mid-brain area. A person with PD will generally appear stiffed or rigid. As the muscle strength becomes low in PD, it affects the articulation process, leading to la ack of coordination in motor-speech functioning. This may result in poor prosody and the onset of dysarthria. There are several non-motor symptoms also associated with PD. Some of them include anosmia or hyposmia, declining cognitive ability, depression, sleep dysfunction, psychosis and so on. These heterogeneous symptoms make PD a complex disorder to diagnose. The exact cause of PD is still unknown. It is believed that genetics, environmental factors such as interaction with harmful pesticides or continuous close contact with certain metals, and other biological factors play a combined role in the arousal of the disease.

There is no standard test available for detection of PD. Doctors carefully weigh symptoms, the medical history of the patient, his/her family history and other factors before coming to a final conclusion. Doctors generally conduct a physical examination at first. In some cases, neuro-imaging tests are performed, which are also known as single-photon emission computed tomography (SPECT) to access the status of dopaminergic neurons. There are disease rating scales designed to assess the person for prodromal PD. For example, the Unified Parkinson's Disease Rating Scale (UPDRS) is a universally accepted scale to monitor PD disability and its severity level increases as the time passes. Also, histological studies of cerebrospinal fluid (CSF) to check the level of α-synuclein in Lewy bodies are performed to confirm the diagnosis process, though the invasive nature of this method makes it not suitable in most clinical environments [21].

Until now, no curative measure for PD is available. Treatments are often administered to provide relief to patients by easing their symptoms. An oral course of Levodopa is the most common form of medication used to maintain the level of dopamine. It greatly helps in reducing symptoms like tremors and bradykinesia. Along with that, physical, occupational and speech therapies are also given to PD subjects. Physical therapy may help in movement issues and setting the gait of the patient right. Occupational therapies improve the everyday activity of the patients while addressing their fine motor skills. Speech therapy may be helpful to tackle dysarthria and other linguistic issues caused by the PD. In some cases, a surgical option is also possible, known as deep brain simulation

(DBS). In this procedure, an electrode is planted in one or both sides of the brain, which improves tremors, fluctuating motor response and dyskinesia. For surgical treatment, the patient must be free of any other form of complication and should respond robustly to Levodopa medication. However, none of the above treatment procedures would guarantee a complete or very long-term remedy for PD.

11.4.1 Parkinson's Disease Prognosis and Measurement Rating Scales

There are two popular scales for the assessment of PD: the HY scale (named after its inventors Hoehn and Yahr) and the Unified Parkinson's Disease Rating Scale (UPDRS).

11.4.1.1 HY Scale

According to this scale, the progression of PD is divided into five different stages [22]:

Stage I: In this stage, the PD symptoms are mild enough and are even difficult to be diagnosed by the clinician. Usually, the symptoms appear on one side of the body, and include mild tremor, stiffness and slow movements.

Stage II: The symptoms propagate on both sides of the body. Loss of facial expression and slow blinking are prominent in stage II. Along with that, speech abnormalities may arise, resulting a slurred voice. Also, pain in the neck or back may appear in some cases.

Stage III: Loss of balance can be seen in this stage. The intuitive functions of the body for sudden involuntary changes to adjust during daily activity become compromised and patient often falls during this stage. The disease can clearly be diagnosed when the patient has reached stage III.

Stage IV: The patient becomes dependent and requires assistance to perform some of the daily activities of life. The onset of stage IV comes with partial paralysis of the person.

Stage V: This is the most advanced stage of PD. People are restricted to a bed or a wheelchair. The risk of falling is associated even when the patient tries to stand on his/her own. Hallucinations and delusions are also experienced by people in this stage.

11.4.1.2 UPDRS Scale

The UPDRS scale observes the individual traits of the person [23]. It has four major sections. Each section includes several conditions on the basis of which the assessment is done. Scores are given to each condition in the range of 0–4, where zero indicates no abnormal condition and four indicates severe abnormal condition. Hence, a total score of 199 points towards total disability, whereas a zero score means no disability. The four major sections of UPDRS with some of their important subparts are:

1. Executive Functions, behavioural analysis
   a. Whether forgetting things, addresses, names and so on.
   b. Hallucination/delusions issues

    c. Anxiety

    d. Emotional detachment

    e. Sleep problems

    f. Constipation/urinary problems

    g. Pain and sensation

2. Daily life activities

    a. Trouble in bathing or brushing teeth.

    b. Need assistance for getting dressed, fastening buttons of shirt, sleeves

    c. Difficulty in food chewing or swallowing

    d. Turning in bed, getting in/out of bed

    e. Trouble in doing hobbies

3. General motor functions

    a. Speech problems/dysarthria

    b. Slowness in moment

    c. Tremor

    d. Gait coordination

    e. Posture stability

    f. Stiffness

4. Other motor complications

    a. Abnormal muscle movement, that is, dyskinesia, time period with dyskinesia

    b. Motor fluctuation

11.4.2 INVOLVEMENT OF DIGITAL TECHNOLOGIES FOR DETECTION AND MONITORING OF PD

Advancements in technologies can be seen in various healthcare protocols for detecting and monitoring of various ailments. Popular examples in this regards are electrocardiogram (ECG), magnetic resonance imaging (MRI), electroencephalogram (EEG), electromyogram (EMG) and so on, used widely to record and monitor biomedical images and electrophysiological signals from the human body. These data are observed by both human (clinician) and machine-level experts (artificial intelligence). Particularly, for the case of PD, the Internet of Things (IoT) embedded with wearable sensors and other digital platforms have been proven greatly helpful to track the motion disturbances that occur during the disorder period.

Remote observations of motor functions and the storing important inferences and symptoms using virtual data management system and mobile networking enable healthcare providers to access the patient's current condition and administer or change medications while sitting in a distant location [24]. Technology like iMotor, equipped with a biometric sensing environment, performs motor function tests to assess the score of a person susceptible to muscle motion disorders like Parkinson's [25].

All these mechanisms require an end point physician to diagnose or mark the trajectory of the disease. Many times, the clinician's jobs are made easy and accurate by the application of machine-learning and computer-aided-diagnosis (CAD), where, the end device may be a computer with an in-built programme to do a task. The advantage of the CAD system is that a second opinion about a diagnosis can immediately be

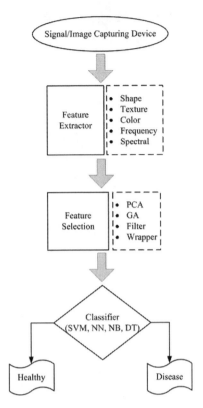

FIGURE 11.2 Generalized block diagram of CAD system. Acronym: PCA = Principle Component Analysis, GA = Genetic Algorithm, SVM = Support Vector Machine, NN = Neural Network, NB = Naive Bayes, DT = Decision Tree.

drawn, thus saving time and extra cost. The basic building blocks of any generalized CAD system are shown in Figure 11.2.

First, the model needs to be trained with the help of samples, for which true labels or ground truths are available. This ground truth is generally given by an expert physician in that area of expertise upon the diagnosis of the person. During the training process, the model is given the input samples' signal or image features and their true class label. The CAD model then tries to develop a relationship between the input features and the output class labels. Once a good training accuracy is achieved, the model is then tested with the completely new samples to ensure its faithful performance. If there is any discrepancy between the training and test set accuracies, the model parameters are again tuned. Finally, when tuning is optimized, and the model gives consistent performance over different test sets, the system will ultimately be recruited for the online direct diagnosis of the disease in order to help the clinicians.

The CAD model performance is highly dependent upon the features extracted from the input samples. Also, too many features exert an extra computational burden since a lot of data may be redundant in nature. Therefore, a suitable feature extraction approach is highly recommended. To subsidize irrelevant and redundant parameters, several feature optimization techniques are employed. Optimization techniques reduce the model complexity and prevent it from overfitting, hence, giving a precise and fast operating scenario.

Many state-of-the-art studies have been done by researchers around the world in the area of machine-learning utility for the diagnosis and prognosis of PD. Tsoulos et al. [25] supported the artificial intelligence application to determine PD patients from a group of people.

They applied neural network construction (NNC) in the data collected by a mobile platform (iMotor, Apptomics Inc., Wellesley, MA) for the classification of patients into PD and healthy controls. They highlighted the important features related with the person having PD. Rastegar et al. [26] tracked the progress of PD by measuring cytokines and chemokines in serum for one year as a baseline and comparing it with the clinical outcomes of the next two years by applying machine learning approaches. The performance of the models was compared via calculating mean errors between their system and HY and UPDRS scales predictions. Grover et al. [27] utilized deep learning networks to predict the severity of PD. The telemonitoring voice dataset was used for the study and achieved better accuracy than previous reported studies. The authors from [28] collected the voice data of persons with and without PD through mPower using an iPhone application for the diagnosis of the disease. The openSMILE features were extracted from the voice and several machine-learning schemes applied, with a peak accuracy of 86% obtained.

Again, the speech as a diagnostic signal for PD was used by Karan et al. [29]. The intrinsic mode function cepstral coefficients (IMFCC) were deduced from empirical mode decomposition and its utility checked by considering two different databases. Excellent performance was reported from IMFCC for the classification of PD patients from their healthy counterparts.

As the mechanism of PD is associated with the function of the brain, electrophysiological signals like EEG may also appear as a significant factor to detect and classify PD subjects. Chaturvedi et al. [30] computed relative EEG power in all bands across different regions of brain. The random forest was applied and found that theta power in the temporal region and alpha/theta ratio in the central region are more compelling biomarkers for the detection of PD. The authors from [31] constructed a 13-layer convolutional neural network architecture to avoid the need for conventional measures for PD categorization. They achieved a classification accuracy of 88.25%. Another study, from [32], explored the potential of higher-order spectra from EEG signals to diagnose PD. Higher-order bispectrum features from EEG were obtained and ranked using a t-value. These ranked features were then subjected to a set of classifiers to evaluate the performance with a minimum number of features. They obtained more than 90% accuracy using the SVM classifier.

From the brief discussion of above, it is evident that machine-learning techniques armed with high-performance computational algorithms and online network management tools are playing a significant role in helping healthcare professionals diagnose PD with a minimum margin of error. Further, the machine approaches work on recorded signals or captured images; hence, it is a faster diagnostic platform compared to a human investigator, which is particularly important when the number of patients is large. Also, a machine is free from any human error, which may introduce fatigue while dealing with subjects and inexperience. Also, if records were stored digitally, prognosis can be done easily. New techniques like deep learning can help when huge of data needs to be assessed. Hence, more and more research in the field of CAD models is recommended and still necessary for effective detection and prognosis of a growing number of patients with PD.

11.5   EPILEPSY

Epilepsy is one of the most common neurological illnesses due to a disorder in nerve cells. Recurrent seizure condition in patient confirms the diseases as epilepsy. If there is a confirmation of a reason for epilepsy, like a head injury, asphyxia and so on, then this type of epilepsy is known as symptomatic epilepsy [33]. The other type of epilepsy is known as idiopathic epilepsy. In idiopathic epilepsy, the reason for the epilepsy is unidentifiable. The incidence of this chronic disease is comparably higher in developing countries than developed countries. Millions of people around the world suffer with this disease [34]. This disease makes their social and individual life challenging. An electroencephalogram (EEG)-based clinical approach is the most common and traditional technique used by neurologists to diagnose and detect epilepsy. Since the treatment of epilepsy requires continuous observation through an EEG, it is time-consuming and tedious work for neurologists and consequently degrades their performance. Therefore, the neurologist may not be able to provide treatment services to more patients. These issues can be solved with a machine learning technique-based automatic epilepsy detection system. During the last two decades, huge research studies have been reported worldwide. Some recent related studies are cited below.

11.5.1   RECENT LITERATURES ON EPILEPSY DETECTION

A convolution neural network (CNN)-based epileptic seizure diagnosis and identification system was reported in [35]. In this study, multiclass CNN with 13 layers was developed for epilepsy detection. A classification accuracy of 88.67% was achieved with this proposed model. A novel weighted complex network-based epileptic signals classification model was proposed in [36]. In this research, EEG signals were segmented and clustered into small parts. Further, statistical features were extracted from the cluster of EEG signals. These features were mapped on a weighted network and then network-based local and global features like clustering coefficient, average degree and closeness were extracted. The proposed method used four different classification techniques, support vector machine, k-means, k-nearest neighbour and naive Bayes. An average classification accuracy of 98% was achieved with this method. A significant performance is reported using the 1D-CNN-based epileptic seizure detection model in [37]. In this study, EEG signals were segmented with a fixed slide window and used to make a local decision by multiple 1D-CNN classifiers. This local decision was further used to take a final decision using a majority voting-based algorithm. This model outperformed with an average classification accuracy of 99.1±0.9%. An SVM-based epileptic seizure detection with Hilbert vibration decomposition

(HVD) was implemented in [38]. In this research, Hilbert transform was applied on EEG signals, and HVD-based features were extracted. With these HVD features and SVM classifier, an epileptic seizure detection accuracy of 97.66% was achieved. A bag-of-words approach based on non-linear attributes for an epilepsy detection model was reported in [39]. In this study, wavelet transform-based statistical features were calculated and further clustered with one of the techniques, namely a k-means or expectation–maximization (EM) algorithm. These clustered features were used as new descriptors of EEG signals called bag of words. Finally, a non-linear kernel-based classifier was utilized to classify the bag of words. A classification accuracy of 100% was achieved with SVM, with a radial basis function (RBF). Empirical mode decomposition (EMD) with an ensemble classifier-based epileptic seizure identification approach was proposed in [40]. Normal inverse Gaussian (NIG) parameters from the EMD were extracted as features. An accuracy of 100% was achieved for seizure versus healthy EEG signals classification. A comparative study of classifier performances with wavelet-based statistical features of EEG signals for the epileptic seizure detection process was done in [41]. In this research, a total of 150 features were extracted. Further, three feature selection algorithms, information gain (IG), relief-F (RLF), and correlation (P) algorithms were used to select relevant features from a large feature vector. The performances of 16 classification models for full features and the top 30 features of the three above-mentioned feature selection methods were evaluated in this study. An accuracy of 100% was achieved with only 30 relevant features selected by IG and RLF with a back propagation artificial neural network classifier.

11.5.2 GENERALIZED MACHINE LEARNING MODEL FOR EPILEPSY DETECTION SYSTEM

Figure 11.3 depicts a generalized machine learning model for an EEG-based epileptic seizure identification system. The whole epileptic detection model is divided into two parts with a vertical discontinuous line, as shown in Figure 11.3. Part I is referred to as the training section of the machine learning model. In this section, acquired EEG signals are pre-processed with noise removal techniques like a digital band-pass filter, a notch filter and independent component analysis (ICA). In the next step, features are extracted from pre-processed EEG signals. Wavelet decomposition, statistical features, EMD and HVD are some reported techniques used to extract the features from EEG signals. The short-time Fourier transform (STFT)-based feature extraction process is also reported in recent articles [42]. Feature selection algorithms are used to pick relevant features from a large feature vector in further steps. Feature selection algorithms rank the feature according to specific criteria. In the next step, the machine learning classifier is trained with prime attributes and ground truth. In the learning process of classifier, the supervision is provided by epilepsy disease neurology experts as in the form of ground truth. Finally, the machine learning model is trained and generates learning parameters.

Part II of the model is referred as the testing section of the machine learning model. In this section, live decisions are taken by the epileptic seizure detection system. The pre-processing step is identical to the training section. In the next step, only prime attributes are extracted from the EEG signals. In a further step, the trained model

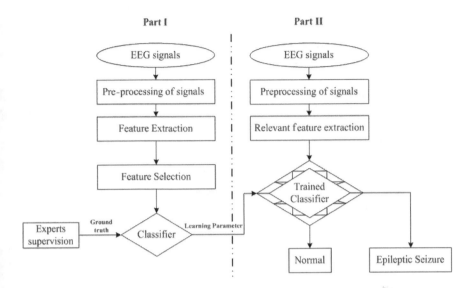

FIGURE 11.3   Machine learning model for epileptic seizure detection system.

takes a decision about the incoming EEG signals according to learning specifications gained during the training process.

In conclusion, epilepsy disease affects approximately 50 million people of the world population. As compared to developed countries, developing countries are more affected with this disease. Medical staffs are also limited in number and there is always a chance of human error during restless treatment. The machine learning-based epileptic seizure detection model may assist the neurologist or medical staff to provide error-free treatment to more patients and improved medical facilities.

11.6   SCHIZOPHRENIA

Schizophrenia (SCZ) is one of the most critical psychiatric disorders. According to a report by the World Health Organization (WHO), approximately 20 million people of the world population suffer from this mental illness [43]. Psychiatrist case studies have reported that this disorder not only tortures the sufferer but also leads nearby persons and family members into surprising trouble [44]. Hallucinations, disorganized speech, attention impairment and delusion are some behavioural and psychotic symptoms of the SCZ patient [45]. Long-term medication is mostly required for treatment in the late detection of this mental anomaly. The severity of SCZ disease is measured using a standard clinical scale, namely Positive and Negative Syndrome Scale (PANSS) [46]. The symptoms of this disease are quite similar to other mental illnesses. Therefore, there is a requirement of good psychiatric experience in treatment. Until now, face-to-face interview-based diagnoses have been performed to detect and provide treatment to SCZ patients. No advanced tools are available to aid the psychiatrist. Hence, there is an extreme need for an intelligent detection and diagnostic tool to identify this disease.

11.6.1 Recent Research

A combination of source- and sensor-level EEG features for machine learning-based SCZ detection was proposed in [5]. In this study, event-related potential based features were used as sensor-level EEG features. A maximum classification accuracy of 88.24% was reported with combined features and an SVM classifier. An EEG signal during visual stimulus for the evocation of an emotion-based SCZ detection system was proposed in [47]. In this research, three different entropy-based attributes from EEG signals were computed for classification. This system was able to classify healthy subjects versus markedly ill into SCZ, and moderate ill versus markedly ill into SCZ with an accuracy of 81.5% and 79.5% respectively. A study on steady-state visual evoked potential (SSVEP) features-based system for classification of bipolar disorder and SCZ was reported in [48]. In this study, features like mean, skewness and kurtosis of SSVEP SNR values were computed. Then, the Fisher scores were computed for all attributes, to rank and select the most relevant features. The highest classification accuracy of 91.3% was achieved by using the k-nearest neighbour (kNN) classifier.

An 11-layer convolution neural network (CNN)-based detection system for SCZ was proposed in [49]. In this research, subject-based and non-subject-based CNN models were proposed for the detection of SCZ. For the subject-based testing model, five convolutions and pooling layer pairs and one fully connected layer were utilised, while in the non-subject-based testing model, four convolutions and pooling layer pairs and three fully connected layers were used. Classification accuracy of 98.07% and 81.26% were achieved for the non-subject-based and the subject-based testing system respectively. A spectral analysis of an EEG signals-based SCZ identification model was reported in [50]. In this research, an overall classification accuracy of 71.43% was achieved with a random forest (RF) classifier. This simple RF-based model was reported to have provided faster response when tested on a regular computer. A deep learning-based SCZ detection system was reported in [51]. In this study, EEG signals were transformed into two-dimensional spectrograms using STFT. Further, classification was done using a convolution neural network (CNN), namely VGG-16, and with a reported classification accuracy of 97%. An article on a kernel SVM-based artificial intelligence system for detection of SCZ disease was reported in [52]. In this research, a wavelet-based EEG rhythm's statistical attributes were extracted from EEG signals. Further, a Mann–Whitney U test was conducted to sort out the statistically significant attributes. These significant features were employed for classification purposes. Classification accuracy of 78.95% and 89.29% were achieved for SCZ versus healthy subjects, and negative symptom (NS) versus positive symptom (PS) SCZ condition respectively.

11.6.2 A Machine Learning Model for Schizophrenia Detection

A generalised supervision model of schizophrenia detection based on EEG and machine learning technique is shown in Figure 11.4. The whole model is divided into two parts, the training part and the test part. In the training part, the first step of the

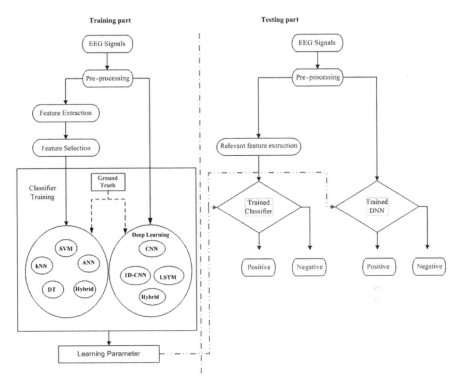

FIGURE 11.4 Machine learning model for schizophrenia detection system.

model is the signal/data acquisition. Here, the EEG modality is used to acquire the brain signals from patients/subjects. Resting signals as well as stimulus-based EEG signals can be used in the detection of SCZ disease. The next and most essential step is the pre-processing of signals. This procedural step removes the unwanted noises captured simultaneously during data acquisition. As depicted in Figure 11.4, further steps are dependent on the selection of the classifier. Feature extraction and selection steps play an important role in traditional classifiers like SVM, kNN, decision tree (DT), artificial neural network (ANN), and hybrid classifier based on these classifiers, whereas there is no requirement for feature extraction and selection steps in deep neural network-based classifiers like CNN, 1D-CNN, (LSTM). The procedures of feature extraction and selection are performed by the deep neural network inside of the layers. In the next step, the selected classifier is trained with training signals and their ground truth decided by experienced psychiatrists. After successful training, the learning parameters are generated. These parameters help the trained classifier to take a decision on unknown signals during testing. The testing part of the model involves taking the initial two steps as we have done in the training stage. The difference is that only relevant features are extracted in the traditional classifier case, while in DNN, the inside layer's learning parameters are decided upon as the important features in the signals. Finally, the trained classifier takes decisions on signals according to the training.

In conclusion, research on the classification of SCZ versus healthy subjects, positive syndrome (PS) versus negative syndrome (NS), and SCZ versus other mental illness are already reported in the literature. Still, there is a need for sufficient research on the machine learning-based SCZ detection system. A machine learning-based SCZ detection system will be helpful in the treatment and diagnosis of SCZ patients and also aid the psychiatrist as a supporting tool.

LEARNING OUTCOMES

At the end of studying this chapter, the students and learners will be able to:

- Explain overview of various neurodevelopmental disorders, such as attention-deficit/hyperactivity disorder (ADHD), Parkinson's disease, epilepsy and schizophrenia
- Elaborate developmental dyslexia and diagnostic methods

REFERENCES

1. Badalà, F., Nouri-mahdavi, K., & Raoof, D. A. (2015). Neurobiology of dyslexia. *Current Opinion in Neurobiology, 30*, 73–78.
2. Shaywitz, S. E., & Shaywitz, B. A. (2008). Paying attention to reading: The neurobiology of reading and dyslexia. *Development and Psychopathology, 20*(4), 1329–1349.
3. Ullah Khan, R., Lee, J., Cheng, A., & Bee, O. Y. (2018). Machine learning and dyslexia: Diagnostic and Classification System (DCS) for kids with learning disabilities. *International Journal of Engeering & Technology, 7*(3), 97–100.
4. Asvestopoulou, T. et al. (2019). DysLexML: Screening tool for dyslexia using machine learning. https://arxiv.org/abs/1903.06274
5. Tamboer, P., Vorst, H. C. M., Ghebreab, S., & Scholte, H. S. (2016). Machine learning and dyslexia: Classification of individual structural neuro-imaging scans of students with and without dyslexia. *NeuroImage Clinical, 11*, 508–514.
6. Pavithran, P. G., Arunkumar, K., Guhan Seshadri, N. P., Kumar Singh, B., Mahesh, V., & Geethanjali, B. (2019). Index of theta/alpha ratio to quantify visual-spatial attention in dyslexics using electroencephalogram. In *2019 5th International Conference on Advanced Computing & Communication Systems (ICACCS)* (pp. 417–422). IEEE. https://doi.org/10.1109/ICACCS.2019.8728482
7. Guhan Seshadri, N. P., Geethanjali, B., & Singh, B. K. (2020). Resting state EEG signal analysis in Indian dyslexic children. In *2020 First International Conference on Power, Control and Computing Technologies (ICPC2T)* (pp. 300–304). https://doi.org/10.1109/ICPC2T48082.2020.9071499
8. *Diagnostic and statistical manual of mental disorders: DSM-5™* (2013). *Diagnostic and statistical manual of mental disorders: DSM-5™* (5th ed.). American Psychiatric Publishing.
9. Faraone, S. V., & Larsson, H. (2019). Genetics of attention deficit hyperactivity disorder. *Molecular Psychiatry, 24*(4), 562–575.
10. World Health Organization. (1993). The ICD-10 classification of mental and behavioural disorders. *Diagnostic Criteria for Research.* www.who.int/classifications/icd/en/bluebook.pdf

11. Minkoff, N. B. (2009). ADHD in managed care: an assessment of the burden of illness and proposed initiatives to improve outcomes. *American Journal of Managed Care, 15*(5 Suppl), S151–S159.

12. Dai, D., Wang, J., Hua, J., & He, H. (2012). Classification of ADHD children through multimodal magnetic resonance imaging. *Frontiers in Systems Neuroscience, 6*, 1–8.

13. Güven, A. et al. (2020). Combining functional near-infrared spectroscopy and EEG measurements for the diagnosis of attention-deficit hyperactivity disorder. *Neural Computing and Applications, 32*(12), 8367–8380.

14. Iannaccone, R., Hauser, T.U., Ball, J., Brandeis, D., Walitza, S., & Brem, S. (2015). Classifying adolescent attention-deficit/hyperactivity disorder (ADHD) based on functional and structural imaging. *European Child & Adolescent Psychiatry, 24*(10), 1279–1289.

15. Ariyarathne, G., De Silva, S., Dayarathna, S., Meedeniya, D., & Jayarathne, S. (2020). ADHD identification using convolutional neural network with seed-based approach for FMRI data. In *Proceedings of the 2020 9th International Conference on Software and Computer Applications* (pp. 31–35). Association for Computing Machinery.

16. Moghaddari, M., Lighvan, M. Z., & Danishvar, S. (2020). Diagnose ADHD disorder in children using convolutional neural network based on continuous mental task EEG. *Computer Methods and Programs in Biomedicine, 197*, 105738. https://doi.org/10.1016/j.cmpb.2020.105738

17. Marvanova, M. (2016). Introduction to Parkinson's disease (PD) and its complications. *The Mental Health Clinician, 6*(5), 229–235. https://doi.org/10.9740/mhc.2016.09.229

18. Nussbaum, R. L., & Ellis, C. E. (2003). Alzheimer's disease and Parkinson's disease. *New England Journal of Medicine, 348*(14), 1356–1364.

19. Tanner, C. M., & Goldman, S. M. (1996). Epidemiology of Parkinson's disease. *Neurologic Clinics, 14*(2), 317–335.

20. Dorsey, E. R. et al. (2007). Projected number of people with Parkinson disease in the most populous nations, 2005 through 2030. *Neurology, 68*(5), 384–386.

21. Atik, A., Stewart, T., & Zhang, J. (2016). Alpha-synuclein as a biomarker for Parkinson's disease. *Brain Pathology, 26*(3), 410–418.

22. Hoehn, M. M., & Yahr, M. D. (1967). Parkinsonism: Onset, progression, and mortality. *Neurology, 17*(5), 427–442.

23. Movement Disorder Society. (2003). The Unified Parkinson's Disease Rating Scale (UPDRS): Status and recommendations. *Movement Disorders, 18*(7), 738–750.

24. Espay, A. J. et al. (2016). Technology in Parkinson's disease: Challenges and opportunities. *Movement Disorders, 31*(9), 1272–1282.

25. Tsoulos, I. G. , Mitsi, G., Stavrakoudis, A., & Papapetropoulos, S. (2019). Application of machine learning in a Parkinson's Disease digital biomarker dataset using neural network construction (NNC) methodology discriminates patient motor status. *Frontiers in ICT, 6*.

26. Ahmadi Rastegar, D., Ho, N., Halliday, G.M., & Dzamko, N. (2019). Parkinson's progression prediction using machine learning and serum cytokines. *npj Parkinson's Disease, 5*(14). https://doi.org/10.1038/s41531-019-0086-4

27. Grover, S., Bhartia, S., Akshama, Yadav, A., & Seeja, K. R. (2018). Predicting severity of Parkinson's disease using deep learning. *Procedia Computer Science, 132*, 1788–1794.

28. Wroge, T. J., Özkanca, Y., Demiroglu, C., Si, D., Atkins, D. C., & Ghomi, R. H. (2019). Parkinson's disease diagnosis using machine learning and voice. In IEEE (Ed.), *2018 IEEE Signal Processing in Medicine and Biology Symposium (SPMB)* (pp. 1–7). IEEE. https://doi.org/10.1109/SPMB.2018.8615607

29. Karan, B., Sahu, S. S., & Mahto, K. (2020). Parkinson disease prediction using intrinsic mode function based features from speech signal. *Biocybernetics and Biomedical Engineering, 40*(1), 249–264.

30. Chaturvedi, M. et al. (2017). Quantitative EEG (QEEG) measures differentiate Parkinson's disease (PD) patients from healthy controls (HC). *Frontiers in Aging Neuroscience, 9*(3). https://doi.org/ 10.3389/fnagi.2017.00003

31. Oh, S. L. et al. (2020). A deep learning approach for Parkinson's disease diagnosis from EEG signals. *Neural Computing and Applications, 32*(15), 10927–10933.

32. Yuvaraj, R., Rajendra Acharya, U., & Hagiwara, Y. (2018). A novel Parkinson's disease diagnosis index using higher-order spectra features in EEG signals. *Neural Computing and Applications, 30*(4), 1225–1235.

33. WHO. (2002). *Epilepsy: A manual for medical and clinical officers in Africa and clinical officers. World Health Organization.*

34. WHO. (2019). Epilepsy. www.who.int/news-room/fact-sheets/detail/epilepsy

35. Acharya, U. R., Oh, S. L. , Hagiwara, Y., Tan, J. H., & Adeli, H. (2018). Deep convolutional neural network for the automated detection and diagnosis of seizure using EEG signals. *Computers in Biology and Medicine, 100*, 270–278. https://doi.org/10.1016/j.compbiomed.2017.09.017

36. Diykh, M., Li, Y., & Wen, P. (2017). Classify epileptic EEG signals using weighted complex networks based community structure detection. *Expert Systems with Applications, 90*, 87–100.

37. Ullah, I., Hussain, M., Qazi, E. ul H., & Aboalsamh, H. (2018). An automated system for epilepsy detection using EEG brain signals based on deep learning approach. *Expert Systems with Applications, 107*, 61–71.

38. Mutlu, A. Y. (2018). Detection of epileptic dysfunctions in EEG signals using Hilbert vibration decomposition. *Biomedical Signal Processing and Control, 40*, 33–40.

39. Martinez-del-Rincon, J. et al. (2017). Non-linear classifiers applied to EEG analysis for epilepsy seizure detection. *Expert Systems with Applications, 86*, 99–112.

40. Hassan, A. R., Subasi, A., & Zhang, Y. (2020). Epilepsy seizure detection using complete ensemble empirical mode decomposition with adaptive noise. *Knowledge-Based Systems, 191*, 105333. https://doi.org/10.1016/j.knosys.2019.105333

41. Mandal, S., Thakur, M., Thakur, K., & Singh, B. K. (2021). Comparative investigation of different classification techniques for epilepsy detection using EEG signals. In A. A. Rizvanov, B. K. Singh, & P. Ganasala (Eds.), *Advances in biomedical engineering and technology: Select proceedings of ICBEST 2018* (1st ed.). (pp. 413–424). Springer Singapore.

42. Mandal, S., Thakur, K., Singh, B. K., & Ram, H. (2020). Performance evaluation of spectrogram based epilepsy detection techniques using gray scale features, *Journal of Ravishankar University, 33*(1), 1–7.

43. WHO. (2019). Schizophrenia. www.who.int/news-room/fact-sheets/detail/schizophrenia

44. Manford, M. (1998). An Atlas of Epilepsy. *J Neurol Neurosurg Psychiatry, 65*(1), 139. https://jnnp.bmj.com/content/65/1/139.2

45. Andreasen, N. C. (1982). Negative symptoms in schizophrenia: Definition and reliability. *Archives of General Psychiatry, 39*(7), 784–788.

46. Kay, S. R., Fiszbein, A., & Opler, L. A. (1987). The positive and negative syndrome scale (PANSS) for schizophrenia. *Schizophrenia Bulletin, 13*(2), 261–276.

47. Chu, W. L. , Huang, M. W., Jian, B. L., & Cheng, K. S. (2017). Analysis of EEG entropy during visual evocation of emotion in schizophrenia. *Annals of General Psychiatry, 16*(1), 1–9.

48. Alimardani, F., Cho, J. H. , Boostani, R., & Hwang, H. J. (2018). Classification of bipolar disorder and schizophrenia using steady-state visual evoked potential based features. *IEEE Access, 6*, 40379–40388.

49. Oh, S. L., Vicnesh, J., Ciaccio, E. J., Yuvaraj, R., & Acharya, U. R. (2019). Deep convolutional neural network model for automated diagnosis of schizophrenia using EEG signals. *Applied Sciences, 9*(14), 2870. https://doi.org/10.3390/app9142870

50. Buettner, R., Hirschmiller, M., Schlosser, K., Rossle, M., Fernandes, M., & Timm, I. J. (2019). High-performance exclusion of schizophrenia using a novel machine learning method on EEG data. In IEEE (Ed.). *2019 IEEE International Conference on E-health Networking, Application & Services (HealthCom)* (pp. 1–6). IEEE.

51. Aslan, Z., & Akin, M. (2020). Automatic detection of schizophrenia by applying deep learning over spectrogram images of EEG signals. *Traitement du Signal, 37*(2), 235–244.

52. Kandeger, A., Guler, H. A., Egilmez, U., & Guler, O. (2017). Major depressive disorder comorbid severe hydrocephalus caused by Arnold–Chiari malformation: Does exposure to a seclusion and restraint event during clerkship influence medical students' attitudes toward psychiatry? *Indian Journal of Psychiatry, 59*(4), 520–521 https://doi.org/10.4103/psychiatry.IndianJPsychiatry_225_17

12 Applications and Challenges

LEARNING OBJECTIVES

This chapter aims to cover:

- Importance of machine learning in healthcare sector
- Role of machine learning, specifically in diagnosis of diabetes; neuropathy, drug monitoring, bioinformatics, DNA analysis and digital health records
- Highlighting future research directions

12.1 ROLE OF MACHINE LEARNING IN HEALTHCARE RESEARCH

In modern diagnostics used in the healthcare sector, automation and computer-aided diagnosis (CAD) have dominated the traditional methods and equipment for the examination of various types of medical image modalities used in the diagnosis process for different diseases. Efficient diagnosis results are obtained by using machine learning methods, which are actually used as brain signal processing and assist in achieving optimal diagnosis results [1–3]. The CAD systems used in healthcare employ computer algorithms for the training and learning of medical image modalities, which include computed tomography (CT), magnetic resonance imaging (MCRI), X-ray, electroencephalography (EEG) and so on. These images are captured as raw data and subjected to pre-processing operations using suitable signal processing filters or transforms so that the image data becomes suitable for further analysis and stages of the CAD [3–6].

During Covid-19 pandemic situations, we have seen the use of robots serving medicines and food to patients with the virus who have been admitted to various hospitals. This is a brilliant example of computer machine and machine learning in healthcare [7–9]. The understanding capabilities both in robots and CAD systems are attributed to the learning process, which is facilitated by the suitable machine learning method such as neural network (NN), k-means algorithm, linear regression, clustering, support vector machine (SVM), naive Bayes and so on, [2], [4], [4], [9–20], among which deep learning is seen as the most emerging neural network that can handle a huge amount of data and can perform speedy tasks associated with

DOI: 10.1201/9781003097808-12

CAD in healthcare [15], [19–21]. Breast cancer diagnosis using mammograms and classifiers is suggested in [22], [10], [1] and [3]. The healthcare sector and health informatics perform efficiently using CAD systems that employ modern machine learning methods and artificial intelligence. The advent of deep learning makes it more efficient in terms of handling huge amounts of data and large processing times.

12.2 EFFICIENT DIAGNOSIS OF DIABETES

Diabetes is reported as the most common disease in a large number of people all across the world. The diagnosis and treatment employs machine learning methods in computerized testing and analysis systems. The role of machine learning is very important in classifying various types of deficiencies and stages of diabetes [9], [12], [17], [23–25]. Figure 12.1 shows types of diabetes and their classifications. The glucose level and the insulin level as per the various parameters of patients can be automated using a suitable machine learning method. Figure 12.2 shows different

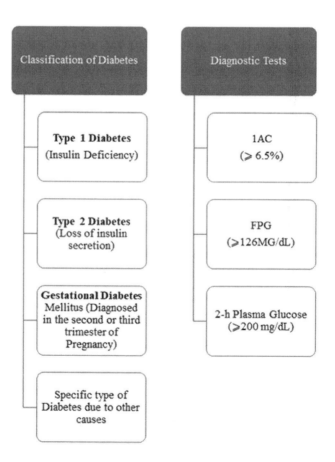

FIGURE 12.1 Classification of diabetes and required tests.

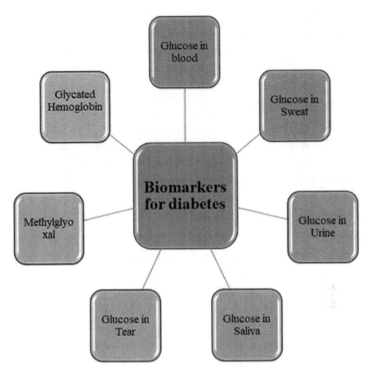

FIGURE 12.2 Biomarkers used in diagnosis of diabetes.

types of biomarkers used in the diagnosis of diabetes, and this complete set-up can also be automated using machine learning methods. Various attributes of analysis such as the glucose level in urine and blood can be monitored and appropriate diagnosis can be suggested to affected patients. In [12], a glucose binding study is presented that employs the support vector machine (SVM) method. Diabetes research uses machine learning and data mining techniques in [13], highlighting supervised, unsupervised and reinforcement learning. Biomarker analysis and prediction was simplified by using machine learning techniques, augmenting the performance of data mining techniques. Ensemble and feature learning in [26] were used in predicting cardiovascular and diabetes diseases, implemented as a data-driven approach. The SVM and logistic regression methods are used for the classification of diabetic and non-diabetic persons. Machine learning methods improve the performance of classification significantly. In several other studies, [27], [28], [9], [29], [4], [25] and [17], diabetes research has been investigated using machine learning methods.

12.3 NEUROPATHY

Neuropathy is a disease involving the damage or dysfunction of nerves in some parts of the body [6], [8], [14], [19], [23], [29–31]. CAD-based systems equipped with AI and machine learning can assist physicians in providing better diagnosis results for this disease. In [19], diabetic neuropathy employs AI for improved classification of nerve disorders. In [30], peripheral neuropathy uses machine learning in the process of chemotherapy. A pain research study in [32], focuses on structure detection and classification using symbolic and sub-symbolic methods. Support vector machine (SVM) is used in diabetic neuropathy in [31] for predictive classification in terms of accuracy and precision. Neuropathy approaches using machine learning were investigated in many studies, and a few of them are reported here that use machine learning in [23], [14] and also [6]. Neuropathy and its automated analysis has become accurate, producing fast and efficient classification results by using machine learning methods.

12.4   DRUG MONITORING

In drug research and monitoring, machine learning and computer vision play a significant role in deciding the proportions and doses of different types of drugs [30], [33], [34]. Right from a sample collection to analysis of results and reporting, the system can work efficiently and produce accurate results in various types of drug discovery-based research. One such scenario has been highlighted in Figure 12.3, which includes the major stages involved in the drug monitoring process. The drug analysis and discovery utilizing machine learning helps in:

- Pre-processing of data and samples
- Feature extraction and selection
- Classification
- Post-processing and applications of analysis

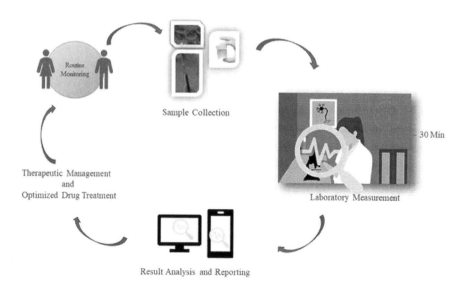

FIGURE 12.3   Drug monitoring and analysis.

12.5 BIOINFORMATICS

Bioinformatics is actually a multidisciplinary field of research and study that involves several major domains, namely biology, mathematics, chemistry, physics, statistics, software engineering, computer science and so on [12], [15], [33], [35]–[37]. Few major domains are shown in Figure 12.4. In working with these domains, there are issues and challenges when implementing various components of an individual domain. Figure 12.5 shows some important issues reported in bioinformatics-based research, which are listed below:

- Big data issues
- Multi-functionality
- Data integrity and security
- Need for multidisciplinary knowledge
- Software design issues
- Accuracy and response time
- Data redundancy

There are numerous tools used in order to simplify and address some major issues that can be seen in Figure 12.6.

There are a number of research contributions and studies on the role of machine learning in the bioinformatics field. We have considered a few important studies among them, which are reported in this section. Predictive and robust modelling was

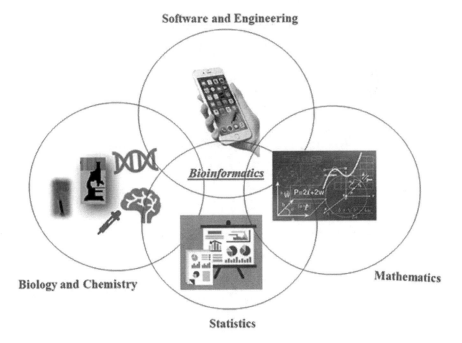

FIGURE 12.4 Different domains of bioinformatics.

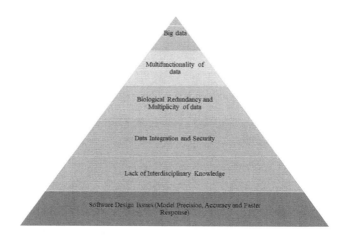

FIGURE 12.5   Various issues in bioinformatics.

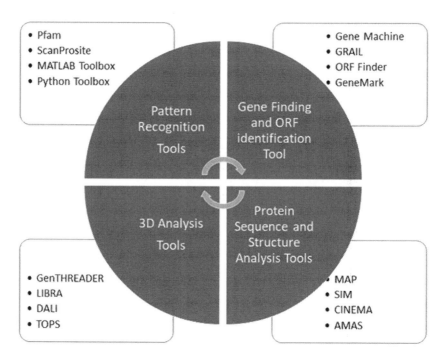

FIGURE 12.6   Tools used in analysis process.

presented in [35], where computational biology and its components were explored using the swarm intelligence concept and machine learning. The comparative analysis employed in this study suggests that robustness is a challenging task, but it can be investigated by comparing a number of machine learning methods tested over the same datasets and similar parameters. In [37], deep learning is used for a bio-informatics and computational biology study. A convolutional neural network (CNN) is presented for the implementation of bioinformatics applications and compared with ordinary machine learning methods. In [33], assessment of predictive accuracy is evaluated for conventional and deep machine learning methods. The techniques were tested over a few important datasets and scoring was checked for measuring the impact of the performance of machine learning methods used in this study. Machine learning for genomic medicine is presented in [38] with an extensive comparative analysis and review of computational issues and datasets of genomics. Deep learning is suggested as an optimal method of machine learning in the analysis of genomics for gene expression, protein binding, computational biology and genome biology.

12.6 DNA ANALYSIS

Analysis of DNA is a complex process that involves huge complexity in computation and implementation, but the advances in machine learning have simplified this area of biological and medical research also [36], [38]. Figure 12.7 depicts some applications

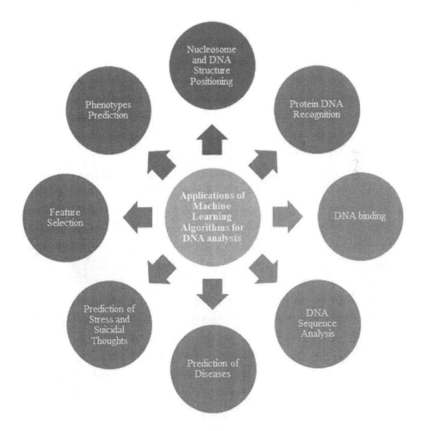

FIGURE 12.7 DNA analysis using machine learning.

of machine learning in various areas of DNA analysis. This includes feature selection, feature extraction, protein synthesis, disease prediction and so on. In [36], DNA barcoding is implemented using machine learning that helps in identifying plants and animals on the basis of sequences and barcodes. A number of features were extracted and subjected to a neural network for classification.

12.7 DIGITAL HEALTH RECORDS

In the age of modern diagnosis usage, a lot of medical data and records pose a big challenge that is addressed by digital health records [9], [13], [26] and [29]. However, the huge amount of data involves complexity and dimensionality, which is solved by an expert system employing AI and machine learning techniques. Figure 12.8 shows few major components of digital health records used in the modern diagnostics and healthcare sector. In [15], deep learning is used in health informatics applications in which the entire health-related information is managed. The CNN and recurrent neural networks (RCN) are used in medical informatics to deal with the following:

- Data complexity issues
- Multimodal data and its challenges
- Lack of incredible results
- Overcoming the limitations of conventional neural network
- Delay in diagnosis and treatment processes

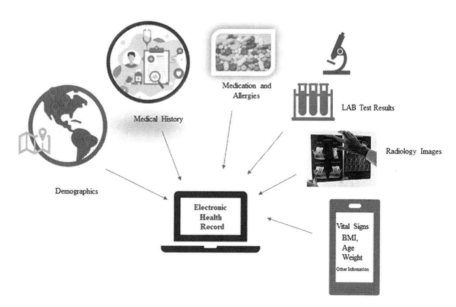

FIGURE 12.8   Electronic health records.

12.8   FUTURE RESEARCH CHALLENGES

Future research directions are mainly towards optimization of various stages and learning impact in healthcare applications. In [39], multitask learning and logical regression are used to augment the performance of existing classifiers and feature extractors. Protein loop modelling employed in several diagnostics and drug discovery uses a novel deep learning [16] which makes predictions of the protein structure. Modern research on cognitive science using machine learning aims at exploring assessment of the cognitive ability of the human brain, and one such study using deep learning is highlighted in [21]. A similar study for cognitive ability assessment was implemented by using deep learning in [20], which reports the abilities of persons for different age groups, gender and so on. In a study of stress and hypertension also, machine learning methods are used. A few major studies on using these various types of machine learning, and including deep learning, are reported in [40], [18], [2], [24], [7] and [41]. In an optimization study of cognitive assessment [42], the performance improvement of classification was emphasized. The future scope of research lies in all-time challenges in the area of machine learning for healthcare and CAD that would aim at overcoming the following:

* Dimensionality of data
* Variability of data
* Diagnosis results are subjective in many cases
* Robustness
* High processing and viewing time

LEARNING OUTCOMES

After studying this chapter, the students will be able to:

* Explain the role of machine learning in healthcare and CAD systems
* Elaborate the applications of machine learning in the analysis and diagnosis of various medical image modalities

REFERENCES

1.   Patel, B. C., Sinha, G. R, & Soni, D. (2019). Detection of masses in mammographic breast cancer images using modified histogram based adaptive thresholding (MHAT) method. *International Journal of Biomedical Engineering and Technology, 29*(2), 134–154. https://doi.org/10.1504/IJBET.2019.097302

2.   New, A., & Bennett, K. P. (2020). A precision environment-wide association study of hypertension via supervised cadre models. *IEEE Journal of Biomedical and Health Informatics, 24*(3), 916–925. https://doi.org/10.1109/JBHI.2019.2918070

3.   Patel, B. C., & Sinha, G. R. (2014). Abnormality detection and classification in computer-aided diagnosis (CAD) of breast cancer images. *Journal of Medical Imaging and Health Informatics, 4*(60), 881–885. https://doi.org/10.1166/jmihi.2014.1349

4.   Ijaz, M. F., Alfian, G., Syafrudin, M., & Rhee, J. (2018). Hybrid prediction model for type 2 diabetes and hypertension using DBSCAN-based outlier detection, Synthetic

Minority Over Sampling Technique (SMOTE), and random forest. *Applied Sciences, 8*(8). https://doi.org/10.3390/app8081325

5. Bhonsle, D., Kumar Chandra, V., & Sinha, G. R. (2018). De-noising of medical images using combined bivariate shrinkage and enhanced total variation technique. *i-manager's Journal on Electronics Engineering, 8*(4), 12–18. https://doi.org/10.26634/jele.8.4.14426

6. Abawajy, J., Kelarev, A., Chowdhury, M. U., & Herbert, F. J. (2016). Enhancing predictive accuracy of cardiac autonomic neuropathy using blood biochemistry features and iterative multitier ensembles. *IEEE Journal of Biomedical and Health Informatics, 20*(1), 408–415. https://doi.org/10.1109/JBHI.2014.2363177

7. Fitriyani, N. L., Syafrudin, M., Alfian, G., & Rhee, J. (2019). Development of disease prediction model based on ensemble learning approach for diabetes and hypertension. *IEEE Access, 7,* 144777–144789. https://doi.org/10.1109/ACCESS.2019.2945129

8. Salahuddin, T., Al-Maadeed, S. A. , Petropoulos, I. N., Malik, R. A., Ilyas, S. K., & Qidwai, U. (2019). Smart neuropathy detection using machine intelligence: Filling the void between clinical practice and early diagnosis. *Proceedings of the 3rd World Conference on Smart Trends in Systems, Security and Sustainability,* WorldS4 2019, 141–146. https://doi.org/10.1109/WorldS4.2019.8904015

9. Abhari, S., Kalhori, S. R. N., Ebrahimi, M., Hasannejadasl, H., & Garavand, A. (2019). Artificial intelligence applications in type 2 diabetes mellitus care: Focus on machine learning methods. *Healthcare Informatics Research, 25*(4), 248–261. https://doi.org/10.4258/hir.2019.25.4.248

10. Patel, B. C., & Sinha, G. R. (2015). Gray level clustering and contrast enhancement (GLC–CE) of mammographic breast cancer images. *CSI Transactions on ICT, 2*(4), 279–286. https://doi.org/10.1007/s40012-015-0062-z

11. Sedaghat, N., Fathy, M., Modarressi, M. H., & Shojaie, A. (2018). Combining supervised and unsupervised learning for improved mirna target prediction. *IEEE/ACM Transactions on Computational Biology and Bioinformatics, 15*(5), 1594–1604. https://doi.org/10.1109/TCBB.2017.2727042

12. Ranganarayanan, P., Thanigesan, N., Ananth, V., Jayaraman, V. K. & Ramakrishnan, V. (2016). Identification of glucose-binding pockets in human serum albumin using support vector machine and molecular dynamics simulations. *IEEE/ACM Transactions on Computational Biology and Bioinformatics, 13*(1), 148–157. https://doi.org/10.1109/TCBB.2015.2415806

13. Kavakiotis, I., Tsave, O., Salifoglou, A., Maglaveras, N., Vlahavas, I., & Chouvarda, I. (2017). Machine learning and data mining methods in diabetes research. *Computational and Structural Biotechnology Journal, 15,* 104–116. https://doi.org/10.1016/j.csbj.2016.12.005

14. Corpin, R. R. A. et al. (2019). Prediction of diabetic peripheral neuropathy (DPN) using plantar pressure analysis and learning models. *2019 IEEE 11th International Conference on Humanoid, Nanotechnology, Information Technology. Communication and Control, Environmental, and Management HNICEM 2019.* https://doi.org/10.1109/HNICEM48295.2019.9072889

15. Ravi, D. et al. (2017). Deep learning for health informatics. *IEEE Journal of Biomedical and Health Informatics, 21*(1), 4–21. https://doi.org/10.1109/JBHI.2016.2636665

16. Nguyen, S. P., Li, Z., Xu, D., & Shang, Y. (2019). New deep learning methods for protein loop modeling. *IEEE/ACM Transactions on Computational Biology and Bioinformatics, 16*(2), 596–606. https://doi.org/10.1109/TCBB.2017.2784434

17. Swapna, G., Vinayakumar, R., & Soman, K. P. (2018). Diabetes detection using deep learning algorithms. *ICT Express, 4*(4), 243–246. https://doi.org/10.1016/j.icte.2018.10.005

18. Wu, J. H. et al. (2019). Risk assessment of hypertension in steel workers based on LVQ and Fisher-SVM deep excavation. *IEEE Access, 7*, 23109–23119. https://doi.org/10.1109/ACCESS.2019.2899625

19. Williams, B. M. et al. (2020). An artificial intelligence-based deep learning algorithm for the diagnosis of diabetic neuropathy using corneal confocal microscopy: a development and validation study. *Diabetologia, 63*(2), 419–430. https://doi.org/10.1007/s00125-019-05023-4

20. Sinha, G. R. (2017). Study of assessment of cognitive ability of human brain using deep learning. *International Journal of Information Technology, 9*(3), 321–326. https://doi.org/10.1007/s41870-017-0025-8

21. Sinha, G. R., Srujan Raju, K., Patra, Raj Kumar, Aye, Daw Win, & Khin, Daw Thuzar. (2018). Research studies on human cognitive ability. *International Journal of Intelligent Defence Support Systems, 5*(4), 298–304. www.inderscienceonline.com/doi/abs/10.1504/IJIDSS.2018.099891

22. Patel, B. C. & Sinha, G. R. (2012). Energy and region based detection and segmentation of breast cancer mammographic images. *International Journal of Image, Graphics and Signal Processing, 4*(6), 44–51. https://doi.org/10.5815/ijigsp.2012.06.07

23. Agurto, C., Barriga, S., Burge, M., & Soliz, P. (2015). Characterization of diabetic peripheral neuropathy in infrared video sequences using independent component analysis. *IEEE International Worshop on Machine Learning for Signal Processing MLSP, 2015*(November), 1–6. https://doi.org/10.1109/MLSP.2015.7324362

24. Mini, G. K., Sarma, P. S., Priya, C., & Thankappan, K. R. (2020). Control of hypertension among teachers in schools in Kerala (CHATS-K), India. *Indian Heart Journal,* no. xxxx, 6–10. https://doi.org/10.1016/j.ihj.2020.06.005

25. Li, Y., Li, H., & Yao, H. (2018). Analysis and study of diabetes follow-up data using a data-mining-based approach in new urban area of Urumqi, Xinjiang, China, 2016–2017. *Computational and Mathematical Methods in Medicine, 2018.* https://doi.org/10.1155/2018/7207151

26. Dinh, A., Miertschin, S., Young, A., & Mohanty, S. D. (2019). A data-driven approach to predicting diabetes and cardiovascular disease with machine learning. *BMC Medical Informatics and Decision Making, 19*(1), 1–15. https://doi.org/10.1186/s12911-019-0918-5

27. Farran, B., AlWotayan, R., Alkandari, H., Al-Abdulrazzaq, D., Channanath, A., & Thanaraj, A. (2019). Use of non-invasive parameters and machine-learning algorithms for predicting future risk of type 2 diabetes: A retrospective cohort study of health data from Kuwait. *Frontiers in Endocrinology (Lausanne), 10*(September), 1–11. https://doi.org/10.3389/fendo.2019.00624

28. Makino, M. et al. (2019). Artificial intelligence predicts the progression of diabetic kidney disease using big data machine learning. *Scientific Reports, 9*(1), 1–9. https://doi.org/10.1038/s41598-019-48263-5

29. Dagliati, A. et al. (2018). Machine learning methods to predict diabetes complications. *Journal of Diabetes Science and Technology, 12*(2), 295–302. https://doi.org/10.1177/1932296817706375

30. Bloomingdale, P., & Mager, D. E. (2019). Machine learning models for the prediction of chemotherapy-induced peripheral neuropathy. *Pharmaceutical Research, 36*(2), 1–12. https://doi.org/10.1007/s11095-018-2562-7

31. Kazemi, M., Moghimbeigi, A., Kiani, J., Mahjub, H., & Faradmal, J. (2016). Diabetic peripheral neuropathy class prediction by multicategory support vector machine model: a cross-sectional study. *Epidemiology and Health, 38*, e2016011. https://doi.org/10.4178/epih.e2016011

32. Lötsch, J., & Ultsch, A. (2018). Machine learning in pain research. *Pain, 159*(4), 623–630. https://doi.org/10.1097/j.pain.0000000000001118

33. Ashtawy, H. M., & Mahapatra, N. R. (2015). A comparative assessment of predictive accuracies of conventional and machine learning scoring functions for protein-ligand binding affinity prediction. *IEEE/ACM Transactions on Computational Biology and Bioinformatics, 12*(2), 335–347. https://doi.org/10.1109/TCBB.2014.2351824

34. Miranda, A. M., Goulart, A. C., Benseñor, I. M., Lotufo, P. A., & Marchioni, D. M. (2021). Coffee consumption and risk of hypertension: A prospective analysis in the cohort study. *Clinical Nutrition, 40*(2), 542–549. https://doi.org/10.1016/j.clnu.2020.05.052

35. Alves, P., Liu, S., Wang, D., & Gerstein, M. (2018). Multiple-swarm ensembles: Improving the predictive power and robustness of predictive models and its use in computational biology. *IEEE/ACM Transactions on Computational Biology and Bioinformatics, 15*(3), 926–933. https://doi.org/10.1109/TCBB.2017.2691329

36. Ma, E. Y. T., Ratnasingham, S., & Kremer, S. C. (2018). Machine learned replacement of N-Labels for basecalled sequences in DNA barcoding. *IEEE/ACM Transactions on Computational Biology and Bioinformatics, 15*(1), 191–204. https://doi.org/10.1109/TCBB.2016.2598752

37. Tang, B., Pan, Z., Yin, K., & Khateeb, A. (2019). Recent advances of deep learning in bioinformatics and computational biology. *Frontiers in Genetics, 10*(March), 1–10. https://doi.org/10.3389/fgene.2019.00214

38. Leung, M. K. K., Delong, A., Alipanahi, B., & Frey, B. J. (2016). Machine learning in genomic medicine: A review of computational problems and data sets. *Proceedings of the IEEE, 104*(1), 176–197. https://doi.org/10.1109/JPROC.2015.2494198

39. Liang, A., Zhu, L., & Huang, D. S. (2018). Optimization of gene set annotations using robust trace-norm multitask learning. *IEEE/ACM Transactions on Computational Biology and Bioinformatics, 15*(3), 1016–1021. https://doi.org/10.1109/TCBB.2017.2690427

40. Chen, J. B., Wu, K. C., Moi, S. H., Chuang, L. Y., & Yang, C. H. (2020). Deep learning for intradialytic hypotension prediction in hemodialysis patients. *IEEE Access, 8*, 82382–82390. https://doi.org/10.1109/ACCESS.2020.2988993

41. Desai, R., Park, H., Dietrich, E. A., & Smith, S. M. (2020). Trends in ambulatory blood pressure monitoring use for confirmation or monitoring of hypertension and resistant hypertension among the commercially insured in the U.S., 2008–2017. *International Journal of Cardiology: Hypertension, 6*(May), 100033. https://doi.org/10.1016/j.ijchy.2020.100033

42. Mohdowale, S., Sahu, M., Sinha, G. R., & Bajaj, V. (2020). Automated cognitive workload assessment using logical teaching learning-based optimization and PROMETHEE multi-criteria decision making approach. *IEEE Sensors Journal, 20*(22), 13629–13637. https://doi.org/10.1109/JSEN.2020.3006486

Index

A

Artefacts: muscular Artefact, 72; noise, 72; ocular artefact, 72; power line interference, 72; Artificial Neural Network (ANN), 121

Attention-Deficit Hyperactivity Disorder diagnosis, 196; introduction, 195; screening, 196; symptoms, 195; types, 195

B

Bio-signals: electrocardiogram, 65; electroencephalogram, 68; electromyogram, 69; electrooculogram, 69

Bioinformatics, 217

Breast Imaging: benign tumor, 138; malignant tumor, 138; Reporting, 141; Bronchoscopy: biopsy, 181; bronchial lavage, 182

C

Cancer Detection: mammogram, 136; microcalcification, 135

Central tendency, 3

Clustering: FUZZY C-means clustering, 129; K-means clustering, 125

Correlation: pearson correlation, 15; spearman rank correlation, 16

Curve fitting: linear relationship, 14; non- linear relationship, 14

D

Data acquisition: data augmentation, 38; data cleaning, 39; data labelling, 38; pre-processing, 35; Data formats: BDF, 37; DICOM, 36; EDF, 37; GDF, 38; MINC, 36; NIfTI, 36

Decision Tree, 119

Deletion: listwise deletion, 40; pairwise deletion, 40

Diabetes, 214

Digital Health Records, 220

Distribution functions: binomial distribution, 29; normal distribution, 30; poisson distribution, 30

DNA, 219

Drug Monitoring, 216

Dyslexia: behavior, 192; brain imaging, 193; diagnosis, 192

E

Epilepsy: detection, 203; machine learning model for detection, 204: Estimation, 31

F

Feature extraction: statistical feature, 91; texture feature extraction, 78

I

Image enhancement Histogram: equalization, 51; image de-noising, 56; segmentation, 59; spatial filtering, 56; transform domain filtering, 58

Image Processing: classification, 146; feature extraction, 143; feature selection, 145; pre-processing, 142; segmentation, 143

Imputation: data imputation, 41; maximum likelihood imputation, 41: multiple imputations, 40

K

K-Nearest Neighbor Classifier, 117

Kurtosis: leptokurtic, 13; mesokurtic, 11; platykurtic, 14

M

Machine Learning: classification, 107; implementation, 108; reinforcement learning, 109: semi-supervised learning, 109: supervised learning, 114; testing, 113; training, 113; unsupervised learning, 109; validation, 113

Medical Image modalities: elastography, 46; magnetic resonance imaging, 47: photoacoustic imaging, 47: positron emission tomography, 46: radiographies, 46; tomography, 47; ultrasound imaging, 48

Moment Invariants, 100

N

Naïve Bayes Classifier, 114

Neurodevelopmental Disorders: diagnosis, 191; disorder, 191

Neuropathy, 215

Normalization, 102

P

Parkinson's Disease: HY scale, 199; measurement, 199; monitoring, 200; prognosis, 199; rating scales, 199; UPDRS Scale, 199

Pulmonary Disease: detection, 171; diagnosis, 174; laboratory tests, 180: obstructive lung

disease, 172: pulmonary disorders, 171:
pulmonary function test, 182: restrictive lung
disease, 173

R

Random experiment, 24
Random Forest Classifier, 121
Random variable, 28
Regression: linear regression, 18; regression
coefficients, 19

S

Schizophrenia: detection, 205; machine learning
model for detection, 206: Sickle Cell Disease:

clinical complications, 156; management, 168;
severity detection, 155
Statistical significance, 6
Support Vector Machine (SVM), 115

T

Texture feature: co-occurrence matrices, 82;
difference statistics, 87; fractal dimension, 93;
grey-level, 82; neighborhood grey-tone, 88;
run-length, 96; spectral measure, 95

X

X-ray: ionizing radiation, 175; radioisotopes,
176